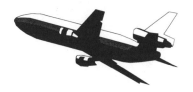

PLANE TRUTH

*Tips for Combating
the Health and Safety Perils of Flying*

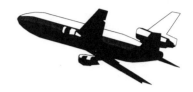

PLANE TRUTH

Tips for Combating
the Health and Safety Perils of Flying

by Riki Stevens,
Ralph Luciani, D.O., Ph.D.,
and Richard Mahler

NEW HORIZON PRESS   **Far Hills, New Jersey**

Requests for permission should be addressed to:
New Horizon Press
P.O. Box 669
Far Hills, NJ 07931

Stevens, Riki, and Ralph Luciani, D.O., Ph.D., and Richard Mahler
    Plane Truth : Tips for combating the health and safety perils of flying

Library of Congress Catalog Card Number: 93-61689

ISBN: 0-88282-094-X (pb)
New Horizon Press

Manufactured in the U.S.A.

1998 1997 1996 1995 1994 / 5 4 3 2 1

Dedication

This book is dedicated to the memory of Lisa Yates, who spent her Pan American Airlines flying career negotiating for the health and safety of fellow flight attendants and the flying public.

Perhaps the most profound statement Lisa made on behalf of the frequent flyer was to the Senate Aviation Subcommittee in the capacity as Director of Health and Safety of the Independent Union of Flight Attendants:

"Since it appears that we are unable to enforce the ozone standards (no monitoring devices on board), how are we to enforce #14 CFR Part 252, *Smoking Aboard Aircraft*, 'Banning smoking when aircraft ventilation is *not* adequate'? Does 'adequate' mean:

- *Adequate to sustain life*—this is, all cabin occupants have physically survived the flight; or
- *Adequate to sustain comfort*—that is, all cabin occupants state they feel no unpleasant physical sensations; or
- *Adequate to sustain health*—that is, they can state they appear to be free of symptoms associated with upper respiratory infections, etc.

Adequate is so general that any attempt at enforcement of even a minimal comfort standard would become difficult."

Contents

Acknowledgments

Gratitude is expressed to the following people who have helped with and given technical and moral support toward completion of this book: Edward T. Bramlitt, Ph.D.; Karen Bramlitt; Barbara and Alvaro Cardona-Hine; Pamela Kent Demers; Elliot Dick, Ph.D.; Susan Fernandez; Michael N. Emmerman; flight attendant Sheryn Frazier; aviation medicine expert Gary Ferris; Dr. John Gofman; Abram Hoffer, Ph.D.; Daniel Holley, Ph.D; Paul A. Hummel, D.C.; Phoebe Hummel, nutrition counselor; Senator Daniel Inouye; Senator Nancy Kassebaum; Mike King; Betty Lind; air safety expert C.O. Miller; Larry Miller, Ph.D.; Rep. Norman Mineta; Captain William Price; Rep. Pat Schroeder; Lynn Stephenson; former Eastern Airlines Captain Steve Stephenson; consumer advocate Chris Witkowski; the flight attendants and pilots who shared their experiences, and the friends and neighbors who were such patient listeners. Special thanks to agents Ruth Aley, Maxwell Aley, and Clark Kimball, who have shown enthusiasm and support from the beginning.

Finally, I wish to acknowledge that the title of this book, *Plane Truth,* was first used in a series of 1989 aviation-related articles written by Robert Kuttner and appearing in *The New Republic.* I thank the magazine's editors for granting me permission to use the title.

MY STORY

"For my part, I travel not to go anywhere, but to go. I travel for travel's sake. The great affair is to move."
—Robert Louis Stevenson

When I started my career as a flight attendant with Continental Airlines, I wanted to travel widely and looked forward to the time off between flights as a chance to satisfy an insatiable curiosity about other people, particularly native tribes.

The job seemed the perfect way to meet my needs. Little did I know what the long-term costs of such a career would be.

I began studying the relationship between flying and health after transferring off an assignment accompanying U.S. soldiers to Viet Nam. My fellow Continental crew members and I had never worked overseas flights until a Military Air Command contract began scheduling commercial carriers on transpacific troop shuttles. As our period of duty lengthened, we found ourselves flying longer hours at higher altitudes than we had experienced previously. We changed time zones as many as twelve times in a single month. Our fatigue was constant and our resistance to disease fell very low. Within eighteen months my own previously good health had completely disintegrated.

I switched back to short-range domestic flights and began to haunt specialty food stores in search of natural methods for repairing my health. It was about six months before I saw positive changes, which I attributed to a healthier lifestyle, fewer time zone changes, and much less stress. I subsequently alternated between domestic and overseas assignments. The international flying always proved to be a health detriment for me. I sensed that many other health-influencing factors existed in airplane travel and strived to learn more about them.

I quit flying when Continental Airlines declared bankruptcy and both duty time and working conditions had become intolerable. I had been a flight attendant for nearly 24 years.

It became obvious to me that my previous health problems had not been caused solely by crossing time zones and changing work shifts. The Senate had heard convincing evidence that the air inside jet cabins was lacking in sufficient oxygen and routinely saturated with viruses, bacteria, carbon monoxide, carbon dioxide, ozone, nicotine, tar, and countless other harmful substances that were constantly being recirculated.

After becoming seriously concerned about the hazardous flying environment and outraged by a lack of action by responsible parties, I became acquainted with radiation health officer Edward T. Bramlitt, a nuclear sciences consultant and Ph.D. in nuclear physics and nuclear chemistry. I subsequently asked him to help me investigate the possible effects of high-altitude and cosmic radiation on frequent fliers. I was alarmed to learn that radiation was increased enough at flight altitudes to prompt Dr. Bramlitt to petition the Federal Aviation Administration (FAA), recommending that airline crew members be classified as radiation workers and required to wear sophisticated monitoring devices called dosimeters. These findings were published in the November 1985 issue of the scientific journal *Health Physics*.

Chairman Daniel K. Inouye (D-HI) and his Senate Aviation Subcommittee members have been addressing these and related issues since 1981. Thousands of health-related complaints from fliers and flight crews have been documented before Congress by airline unions, the FAA, and the National Academy of Sciences. Yet despite conscientious efforts on the part of concerned scientists, legislators, airline employees, and private citizens, little has been done to improve conditions aboard aircraft and to alert passengers about the hazards they unknowingly face.

This is how I began my research for a simple book on flying

and health. But I soon encountered facts so disturbing that, with the help of Dr. Bramlitt and nutrition counselor Phoebe Hummel, I decided to write the more detailed and far-reaching *Plane Truth*.

My concern about this subject led me to get in touch with officials of the Independent Union of Flight Attendants, whom I now have advised on health and safety issues for several years. I have served as a panelist at the Aerospace Medical Association (ASMA) meeting in Las Vegas—along with Dr. Bramlitt and a number of distinguished physicians—on a committee investigating the harmful effects of flying on the reproductive functions of female flight attendants. I chaired the Organizational Structure Study Committee for the Stewards and Stewardesses Division of the Airline Pilots Association; I was the local Los Angeles base chair for Continental's flight attendants; I was the master chairperson for all Continental flight attendant bases, which also involved serving on the contract negotiating committee; I served as advisor on the Merger and Grievance Committee for my union; and I was vice-chairman of an El Paso–based flight attendants' union and an advisor on union organization.

Dr. Ralph Luciani, an aviation and space medicine expert as well as a researcher for the National Aeronautics and Space Administration, contributed important medical advice and technical writing assistance to *Plane Truth*. My information also came from U.S. Senate testimony, concerned public officials, health and safety specialists, and such knowledgeable consumer advocates as Chris Witkowsky, director of aviation consumer action for Ralph Nader. However, most of what I know about the health risks of flying has been obtained from flight personnel: cockpit crews and flight attendants. Bear in mind that if you are a frequent flier you may easily fly as often as these airline professionals; therefore, any information in *Plane Truth* that specifically mentions crew members may very likely apply to you.

Plane Truth goes beyond the scare tactics and hyperbole often found in other books that have reported on this subject. Included is a great deal of practical, easy-to-use information on natural and healthy ways to counteract the hazards of flying. My greatest hope is that *Plane Truth* will serve as a trustworthy guide to help you safely navigate our crowded and busy skies.

Chapter 1

FLYING LOW TO FLYING HIGH

How do you feel after completing a long airplane trip? Are you sick to your stomach or abnormally tired? Do you have a headache or are you more thirsty than usual? Do your limbs sometimes tingle with numbness? Do you find that you need time after flying to make major decisions or to recover your stamina? Do you experience problems with mental acuity or physical dexterity? Do you develop colds or sinus problems within a few days of coming home?

If you can identify with any of the symptoms cited above, you are not alone. All are common side-effects of modern commercial air travel. And while individually they may seem like mere annoyances, when experienced collectively they can compound and aggravate existing medical conditions even to the point of death.

An anxious business executive with high blood pressure and advanced heart disease, for example, may rush to make an early morning flight only to find himself (or herself) sitting on a taxiway breathing in toxic fumes while awaiting takeoff. While the plane sits idle, the amount of fresh oxygen circulating inside the cabin can drop below the minimum amount needed by a passenger's body, contributing to the possibility of a heart attack. Once the traveler is airborne, flight attendants immediately begin offering liquor, coffee, and a fatty meal, further increasing a variety of health risks.

This hypothetical scenario is not intended to suggest a direct cause-and-effect relationship between airline travel and heart attacks, but it is true that an already compromised cardiovascular system can easily be aggravated by flight-related stressors. The American Medical Association and other organizations have acknowledged such risks.

In a 1989 report, *The New York Times* cited a three-year study conducted at London's Heathrow Airport confirming 61 sudden deaths of passengers who had just flown long distances. Most of the victims were women over 40 who had a history of thrombosis (blood clots) in deep veins, and 18 percent of the deaths were ascribed to blood clots in the chest. "Men in their forties with no such history were also victims," the report advised.[1]

Yet most of us never think about such potential outcomes when we board an airplane. Instead the experience is a bit like entering a womb. The cabin is an environment purposefully designed to be reasonably comfortable and cozily efficient. Here we are protected, fed, and attended to—from cockpit to tail—by a staff of polite, well-trained experts.

No wonder so many of us choose to fly. As of 1992, more than 510 million passengers[2] took at least one commercial airline trip annually, up from a mere 16.7 million in 1949. In 1992, 10.5 million flights originated in the U.S. alone.[3] These numbers are growing every year, in part because planes are getting bigger and faster. The standard 21-passenger, propeller-driven DC-3 of the 1930s has given way to the sleek, shiny Boeing 747 Jumbo Jet of the 1990s—ferrying as many as 560 passengers each at record speeds and altitudes.

What most of the thousands of people who fly daily do not realize is that the cabins of the modern jets are not simply beautiful, high-tech cocoons, but also metal-fatigued capsules full of stale air, disease, and high concentrations of radiation, ozone, carbon monoxide, and carbon dioxide. Now more than ever, airplanes can—and do—become flying coffins.

This book will try to open your eyes to the many rarely discussed health risks associated with modern air travel and at the same time provide tips on the best ways to minimize or even eliminate such dangers. In the pages that follow, specific hazards will be outlined in some detail. Following these discussions, various coping strategies and courses of public advocacy will be presented. Since flying has become an unavoidable fact of life for many—if not most—citizens of the United States and other industrialized countries, it would be irresponsible to simply admonish you to avoid air travel altogether. My goal is to be as direct and thorough as possible about the health and safety implications of flying, but to allow plenty of room for optimism as well.

It is important to realize that some airlines do a better job than others in looking after their passengers and crew members. This book gives credit where appropriate to carriers that have distinguished themselves in the area of health and safety.

The Consumer Union, a non-profit watchdog group that publishes *Consumer Reports* magazine, conducted a poll of 140,000 of its readers in 1991 and found Alaska Airlines was rated highest in overall customer satisfaction, followed in descending order by Delta, America West, Southwest, Midway [no longer in business], American, United, and Northwest. At the bottom of the scale were four airlines in deep trouble: Continental, Pan Am, Eastern, and Hawaiian. Two of the latter—Pan Am and Eastern—went out of business shortly after the survey was completed. Separate readership polls by *Condé Nast Traveler* magazine have consistently ranked Alaska and American as the best performing airlines, with Piedmont, TWA, and USAir in the bottom of the top ten. A 1993 study by the International Airline Passengers Association concluded that Air India and Avianca (Colombia's airline) had the worst safety record, while American, British Airways, Delta, Lufthansa, SAS and Southwest had the best.[4]

New Planes, New Problems   ✈

Regrettably, with regard to airplanes, technological progress is not necessarily synonymous with safety. The pioneering Douglas DC-3, fondly referred to as the "vomit comet," did not fly high enough to require pressurization. Fresh air entered the cabin through vents above each seat. The amount of oxygen was adequate and any occasional air sickness was due to turbulence, not poor ventilation. However, if these planes flew above their usual 7,000-foot altitude, as they sometimes did to avoid bad weather, passengers and flight attendants would become sleepy and members of the cockpit crew would don their oxygen masks.

In 1952, Great Britain introduced the first Viscount series turboprop aircraft, allowing higher and longer flights. The necessary pressurization meant redirecting air from the engines into air-conditioning packs that supplied the cabin. The first complaints to U.S. airlines concerning adverse health effects due to cabin air quality were registered that same year.[5]

Modern, high-flying jets such as the Boeing 707 brought with them a new set of health problems. These planes, along with the Boeing 747 Supersonic introduced in 1976, began to routinely fly what are termed "polar" flights. By taking short cuts between continents and flying above the North Pole, passengers and crew came into direct contact with concentrated ozone clusters—where the chemical composition of air is radically altered—and potentially cancer-causing radiation from outer space that penetrated the atmosphere.

Research has shown than when the ozone concentration on airliners reaches 0.15 parts per million, there is a measurable increase in the chance of susceptible passengers having bronchopulmonary attacks and other serious health problems.

Inflight Radiation ✈

The higher the altitude, the greater the intensity of natural but potentially harmful radiation one will encounter, including cosmic radiation emanating from the sun and other celestial bodies. The earth's atmosphere serves as a barrier that protects us to a large degree from such radiation when we are on the ground. Still, some harmful radiation will always be encountered. The presence of ultraviolet rays, for example, can cause skin cancer even at sea level. But the risk of these and other radiation-related illnesses increases dramatically as the atmosphere becomes thinner.

Dr. Edward T. Bramlitt, a world-class nuclear scientist

conducting research on high-altitude radiation, believes that flight crews are exposed to doses so intense that they should be officially classified as radiation workers and ordered to wear sophisticated radiation measurement devices called dosimeters. Bramlitt feels crew members should be monitored regularly for cumulative radiation exposure and warned about its possible health consequences. Yet the FAA has denied Bramlitt's 1984 petition for precisely this kind of protection, and both FAA and airline officials have downplayed or ignored such hazards.[6] Although cockpit crew members were required to wear dosimeters beginning in January 1993, cabin crew members are not covered by this government directive. (For further details, see Chapter 5.)

Oversight and Regulation ✈

It is only recently that U.S. government officials and regulatory agencies have begun taking significant interest in passenger health issues within the aircraft cabin. While seat belts, equipment performance standards, and airplane inspection requirements have been a routine part of the air travel industry for decades, surprisingly little attention has been paid to what members of the public have been breathing when they fly.

In 1981, Hawaii's Democratic Senator Daniel Inouye introduced a bill calling for a complete study of airline cabin air quality and its impact on the health and safety of both crew members and passengers. A modified version of this measure became law in 1984 and a research committee of the National Academy of Sciences (NAS) was awarded almost $600,000 to determine whether "air quality on board commercial airliners is hazardous and whether federal standards adequately protect the health and safety of air travelers." Upon completion of the report, the Secretary of Transportation recommended further study. Almost two years later, on September 19, 1986, the Senate Subcommittee on Aviation held hearings to assess the department's findings.

Much of the material in this book is based on the information and testimony presented during this and other government hearings or gathered by regulatory agencies in response to growing awareness of the health hazards associated with air travel.

Among other things, the National Research Council

Committee (NRCC) of the NAS concluded in its 1986 report that "while the Federal Aviation Administration is clearly responsible for air safety, no federal agency has specific statutory responsibility for protecting the health of airline passengers." The NRCC said the FAA may not have authority to deal with some health-related issues and recommended that this area be placed under the purview of a single federal agency, although it did not suggest which one.[7]

It now appears, however, that the FAA has indeed assumed the role of overseeing all matters regarding health and flying. One high-ranking FAA official has publicly declared that only three harmful contaminants exist in an aircraft cabin: carbon monoxide, carbon dioxide, and high-altitude radiation.[8] Each of these widely recognized contaminants will be discussed in the pages that follow, but it is important to recognize that they represent only a handful of the harmful substances passengers routinely encounter on airplanes.

Chapter 2

HOW FLYING AFFECTS YOUR LUNGS, HEART, AND OTHER VITAL ORGANS

Flying is much more hazardous to their health than most people realize, whether they be "frequent fliers," crew members, or occasional travelers. A primary reason for this is the poor cabin air quality and stressful environment of modern jet airliners.

While most long-suffering airline passengers may not realize the magnitude of flying's health-related dangers, they do know that they often don't feel very good during or after their long plane trips. They may attribute their fatigue and listlessness, along with other common side-effects of air travel, to the rigors of a long-distance journey when a more likely cause is the quality of the air they have been forced to breathe.

As much as 70 percent of the air you inhale on an airplane has been recirculated throughout the cabin, and up to 95 percent of the moisture in that recirculated air is other people's sweat and breath. Undetected to the senses lurk high concentrations of ozone, carbon monoxide, carbon dioxide, and other potentially harmful substances.[1]

The problem is that air comes into the aircraft cabin by way of a plane's jet engines. Since jets fly at altitudes at which oxygen is too thin to support life, the outside (ambient) air must be concentrated for human consumption.[2] The result is that passengers are subjected to a controlled environment.

This situation has improved somewhat since 1990, when the Federal Aviation Administration (FAA) banned smoking aboard all U.S. domestic flights. Most foreign carriers and U.S.-originated international flights, however, still allow smoking in the cabin, and many passengers take full advantage. (Northwest Airlines, Air Canada, and Quantas voluntarily prohibit smoking on all of their flights.)

But even without smokers, the air quality in a plane's cabin is often substandard. One flight attendant—a health and safety officer for her airline—noted in Senate subcommittee testimony that "the vague standard for ventilation in the passenger compartment is the same for transportation of hamsters and guinea pigs in a cargo compartment!"[3]

Flying and Your Respiratory System ✈

The aviation industry's air-filtration system has come under much criticism from passengers and flight attendants who have attributed their frequent headaches and respiratory disorders to poor inflight air quality.

Reporter Dan Rather, in a 1984 CBS News television special on the subject, interviewed a flight attendant who was wearing a hood to protect her identity. The woman discussed her medical claim for permanent respiratory damage due to the lack of proper air ventilation in her working environment.[4]

A similar case involved a flight attendant who suffered permanent respiratory damage after flying West Coast–to–Honolulu runs on DC-8s for a year. When outflow valves on the planes she had been flying were checked, they were found to be significantly clogged by residue. Cabin air cannot be properly exchanged with the ambient air when valves are in this condition.[5]

"I never felt as if I were getting enough air," testified a third flight attendant, in an appearance before the Senate's aviation subcommittee. "I developed asthma because of the conditions on the aircraft. My specialist said it was just a very unhealthy environment in general and that those conditions can aggravate bronchial problems."

Keep in mind that some passengers actually log more airborne hours in a year than regularly scheduled flight crews. Unfortunately, statistics on their health experiences and conditions are not as readily available. Testimony in recent aviation hearings along with the rising tide of consumer complaints indicate that problems related to cabin air quality exist for both groups and are actually getting worse. Yet during a June 1993 report airing on CBS, the FAA reiterated its contention that illness cannot be linked to poor in-flight air, despite appeals by a flight attendants' union to improve cabin air quality.[6]

Cabin Air Conditioning Systems ✈

A jet's cabin air conditioning system works very much like the cooling unit in an automobile, with a few important differences. In an airplane, air drawn from the outdoors is first sterilized of biological elements when compression cycles heat it to very high temperatures. Before distribution into the cabin, however, a portion of recirculated air—that is, "used" air from within the cabin—is mixed with "fresh," ambient air. After circulating inside, the air is either remixed with incoming air or released through the outflow (dump) valves.[7]

Bertil Werjefelt, a health activist and president of a Honolulu-based engineering firm called Vision Safe Inc., claims that the primary cause of cabin air pollution and oxygen depletion is poor maintenance of air ventilation systems and the shutdown of air conditioning units (also called "packs") in order to save fuel. Jet airliners have two or more packs, but they may either shut one or more down or operate all of them at low levels as an economy measure.

Cabin Air Pressure ✈

Werjefelt drew raised eyebrows during Senate aviation committee hearings when he contended that cabin air pressure is *routinely* the equivalent of 9,000 feet above sea level, despite the fact that "the FAA states that their current regulations require cabin altitude not to exceed 8,000 feet for [a] pressurized airplane."

When questioned on this point, Werjefelt noted that federal rules call for a warning signal "when the cabin pressure altitude exceeds 10,000 feet." He pointed out that this is only a design regulation and does not mean that pilots actually heed the warning indication: "The [practical] limit, supposedly, is that at 14,000 feet the oxygen masks are automatically deployed. Dropping the oxygen masks is the only indication (by legal requirement) that a passenger would have that the cabin altitude is then 14,000 feet; in other words, almost twice the 8,000 feet referred to be FAA at the hearings."[8]

The National Academy of Sciences (NAS) shares these concerns, stating in a committee recommendation that "systematic measurement of cabin pressure on a representative sample of routine commercial flights would be advisable."[9]

Air Pack Problems ✈

Flight attendants often bear the brunt of corporate decisions to limit the use of air conditioning packs on long-distance flights. One attendant wrote to me about what happened when packs were deliberately kept at a low setting on the United States–to–Hong Kong route.

"We have experienced headaches and upset stomachs because of it," she said. "It's saving fuel; enough, I hear, so we do not have to make a stop in Taiwan. I don't know if this is the idea of the company or the pilots." Explained retired captain Andy Yates at a meeting of the Aerospace Medical Association, "It's the airline management which puts the pressure on cockpit crews [to limit air pack use]."[10]

A concerned flight attendant looked back on one trip this way: "After takeoff I started feeling lightheaded and found myself moving a lot slower than I would have liked to. I was also very forgetful. . . . Five [of my flying partners] said that they didn't feel well. We ran out of aspirin. . . . Everything I did after that trip was very difficult. I had trouble entering pay records in the computer and my walk to the parking lot was exhausting."[11]

According to a 1990 *Seattle Times* article, Alaska Airlines flight attendants working trips from Alaska to California and Arizona on McDonnell Douglas 80-700 jets reported dizziness, nausea, confusion, swollen lymph glands, headaches, blurred vision, vomiting, weakness, and other problems. In some cases these symptoms lasted for weeks. Some passengers reported severe headaches, gasping for air, and "feeling strange," while flight attendants indicate that travelers tended to sleep an unusual amount of time on these flights. Despite attempts to analyze cargo and clean the air vents, the mystery has never been solved by the airline, the plane manufacturer, or the FAA.[12]

The Boeing 727 and other older model planes circulate cabin air after it has been supposedly vented with new air from the outside and conditioned. This process consumes a lot of fuel, however, and some cost-conscious airlines are purchasing newer planes such as the Boeing 767, which are designed to recirculate 50 percent of the air, thus further lessening your chances of breathing enough oxygen.[13]

Reporting on this issue has sometimes been inaccurate. For example, the *New York Times* in June 1993 erroneously stated that the reduction of fresh air occurs only on planes built since the mid-1980s and repeated assertions by airline officials that there is no correlation between cabin air and passenger health, despite contrary evidence. The newspaper also failed to note that poor cabin air has been studied by the U.S. Senate since 1977 but largely ignored by the FAA.[14]

Protective Air Quality Standards ✈

It is logical to ask whether the FAA has specific standards for quality and ventilation inside aircraft cabins. Federal regulations state only that passenger and crew compartments "must be suitably ventilated." An air circulation rate of ten cubic feet per minute per person is required for crew cabins but not passenger areas. This standard is considered the minimum necessary to avoid feelings of stagnation.[15]

One source of information consulted during the Senate Subcommittee on Aviation's hearings was a recognized authority on air quality: the American Society of Heating, Refrigeration and Air Conditioning Engineers (ASHRAE). While ASHRAE has established ventilation standards for a variety of environments, including the commercial airliner cockpit, it has yet to address concerns regarding passenger compartments. ASHRAE cockpit requirements for fresh air ventilation range from about 70 to 155 cubic feet per minute (cfpm), quite a bit more than the FAA's 10 cfpm. By way of comparison, ambient air circulation averages about 50 cfpm in cocktail lounges, 20 cfpm in offices, and 10 cfpm in bank vaults. Suffocation occurs at zero cfpm.

A 1989 study by the U.S. Department of Transportation concluded that carbon dioxide levels in airline cabins "averaged higher than the ASHRAE standard for comfort." An FAA rulemaking was subsequently introduced to adopt the ASHRAE standard.[16]

"The pilot crew, unlike passengers and flight attendants, receive a much higher quality of air through a separate ventilation system," noted Senator Inouye during the aviation subcommittee's hearings. "If it's good enough for the pilots, why don't the passengers receive this air?"

The first class section and cockpit also have better air quality than the larger cabin, in part because there are simply fewer people seated forward. Vision Safe Inc. recommends cabin air circulation of between 35 to 65 cfpm per passenger as a minimum health standard. This takes into account the amount of space available to each person on an airplane, which may be as little as 35 cubic feet. Again, for comparison, some bars with many people smoking still provide more than 100 cfpm of air circulation per occupant.[17]

Airplane prototypes designed by manufacturers usually provide 15 to 20 cfpm of fresh air in the cabin when tested on the ground. In the air, however, there are no monitors on board (other than often faint cabin attendants and sleepy passengers) to determine whether or not even these standards are maintained.

Another important aspect of the problem is that the cabin may contain any proportion of recirculated and fresh air. Often the circulating air is stale, but because fans are turned on an illusion of fresh air intake is created. Fortunately, passengers spend most of their time seated and require less oxygen than busy flight attendants (who have been known to use supplemental oxygen in the cockpit to get through their shifts).

Most of today's large aircraft, such as the McDonnell

Douglas DC-10, Lockheed L-1011, and Boeing 747, utilize three air packs; one to serve the cockpit and first class, and the other two for the rest of the aircraft. The FAA has certified these planes with "Economy Mode" air conditioning systems that allow complete shutoff of one of the packs while cruising.[18] Economy Mode could supply as little as four to eight cfpm of fresh air per person and is permitted on planes occupied at less than maximum capacity. Airlines can interpret this to be the situation if only one seat is empty.

One or more extra air packs are normally shut off by cockpit crews on international flights or domestic flights that are longer than four hours. Policies vary from one airline to another; some claiming that packs are turned back on if so requested by flight attendants or passengers, during meal service, or if there is too much cigarette smoke in the cabin.

Federal air regulations actually allow the Boeing 727, for example, to take off with one pack inoperative and fly that way indefinitely if its plan restricts flight at or below 25,000 feet altitude. If the remaining pack becomes inoperative, the trip can be continued if the cabin pressure is maintained below 10,000 feet. Crew members say this is a common occurence.[19] Under normal circumstances, air packs are not shut down on smaller aircraft in order to conserve fuel. But pilots are sometimes forced to fly with only one operative pack due to mechanical failure of the other, which is supposed to be repaired at the next stop where such maintenance is available. Often this is not done, however, due to a fear of creating flight delays.

Given the risks mentioned previously, it is questionable why airlines would even consider shutting off an air pack voluntarily. But according to Bertil Werjefelt of Vision Safe Inc., it is "because they can save one to three percent in fuel costs by shutting down one of three air packs." In his testimony before the Senate's aviation subcommittee, Werjefelt said, "To increase [fresh air circulation] to 60 or so cubic feet per minute would require the installation of improved or additional equipment. It does not, however, necessarily translate into added weight. Nor does it substantially have to increase the fuel penalty. We are talking about a total addition of [operating expenses that would add] about one dollar to your air fare."[20]

The Economy Class Blues: Air Packs Restricted ✈

As has been noted, there is quite a difference between the amounts of fresh air received by a cockpit crew, first class passengers, and economy class passengers.

Typically, one pack provides air conditioning for the cockpit and front part of the cabin, while the other one or two packs (on jumbo jets) are assigned to the back cabins.

The cockpit and first class ventilation system is capable of providing as much as 250 cfpm of fresh air and regularly supplies 150 cfpm. Meanwhile, back in the coach seats, passengers and flight attendants are breathing as little as seven cubic feet of vented air per minute per person, most of which is recirculated.

Economy passengers have one air vent (referred to as an "eyeball" or "gasper") above each seat, while cockpit crews are provided with four, and first class travelers may have two or more. In jumbo jets, there are two additional large air vents located above the captain and first officer. Closed cockpit doors also help block most cabin pollutants from entering the cockpit.

Oxygen masks above or in front of passenger seats provide no relief, as they are for emergencies and only release when the cabin altitude reaches the equivalent of 14,000 feet of sea level.[21]

Hypoxia ✈

When your body does not receive enough fresh air, the result can be a condition doctor's call "general hypoxia." Hypoxia is caused by a deficiency of oxygen to the brain and can manifest itself as sleepiness, lassitude, fatigue, sensory impairment, headache, respiratory change (or difficulty), vertigo, increased pulse rate, nausea, blueness around the mouth (or fingernails and earlobes), personality change, mental confusion, memory loss, and even a false sense of euphoria. Eyes and inner ears may also be adversely affected, causing tunnel vision and a loss of balance.[22]

Hypoxia especially affects anemic people. At high altitudes, ample blood flow is needed to carry the smaller amount of available oxygen. Oxygen is carried by the hemoglobin in each red blood cell, and iron is an intrinsic part of that molecule. Anemics, who lack iron, cannot build adequate hemoglobin. One cause of anemia, which is common among flight attendants, appears to be frequent flying.

Anemics usually appear pale and tired, and their tongues and palms lack a normal, deep, red color. Other symptoms include a "heavy feeling in the chest, heart flutters, tiring easily, feeling weak (especially in the arms), trembling hands, and the pallid look associated with poor circulation: purplish with whitish areas around the knuckles when fingers are extended."[23]

Carbon Monoxide ✈

Senate testimony indicates that "carbon monoxide contamination levels inside aircraft are five times higher than the maximum allowed under Environmental Protection Agency (EPA) standards for the general population."[24] FAA regulations specify that carbon monoxide levels should not exceed 50 parts per million, the threshold for what is considered hazardous.

Carbon monoxide combines 210 times more readily with hemoglobin than oxygen to produce hazardous carboxyhemoglobin (COHb), a process that increases under low atmospheric pressure. At high concentrations, COHb disrupts the transfer of carbon dioxide and oxygen within the blood.[25] The National Institute of Occupational Safety and Health reports that "flight attendants who smoke have four to seven percent COHb levels flying in a plane pressurized to 7,500 feet and may experience the equivalent of 10 percent COHb at sea level."[26] It can take more than eight hours to detoxify the COHb after a flight, and frequent fliers may never have enough recovery time to detoxify.[27]

Physicians treating frequent fliers and flight attendants often find elevated COHb levels and repeated instances of reduced pulmonary function. Those with existing lung or heart ailments are also known to be adversely affected by this condition.

Carbon Dioxide ✈

Like carbon monoxide, carbon dioxide is a colorless, odorless gas, somewhat heavier than air, which passes out of the lungs during respiration. While it is a product of normal human metabolism, carbon dioxide can cause problems when there is an insufficient exchange of fresh air. On an airplane a lot of people are exhaling carbon dioxide in a confined space. When the cabin contains a large percentage of recirculated air, rather than fresh, there will be more carbon dioxide than can be tolerated in comfort. Elevated levels can be extremely harmful since breathing an excess of only three percent of carbon dioxide is considered hazardous to humans.

Among the effects of carbon dioxide toxicity are skin sensitivity, sweating, headaches, numbness, and general discomfort. When concentrations of the gas intensify, there is an increase in both the rate and depth of breathing. The latter reach twice the normal rate at 3 percent carbon dioxide, at which point there is also likely to be some physical discomfort. As carbon dioxide levels continue to rise, individuals may experience headaches, malaise, fatigue, and sense that the air is obviously stale.[28]

Human respiration is stimulated by acid or alkaline conditions resulting from metabolic processes and various environmental factors (through a very complicated process of checks and balances). A common reaction among airline passengers to respiratory imbalance is hyperventilation (rapid, shallow breathing). When a person "overbreathes," and too much carbon dioxide is exhaled, respiratory alkalosis may result, with subsequent spasms and muscular twitching.[29]

When this is observed aboard an airplane it is usually attributed to anxiety or a fear of flying, but it also may be due to the high levels of carbon dioxide found in the cabin atmosphere.

Dr. Jack Gorman, director of a biological research center, conducted tests which suggest that people may hyperventilate on a plane because they are "hypersensitive to carbon dioxide, and what makes them hyperventilate is an attempt to keep the carbon dioxide levels low. In effect, the hyperventilation is an adaptation to an abnormal receptive sensor in the brain to carbon dioxide."[30]

Excess levels of carbon dioxide can be extremely harmful. Inhaling as little as one percent carbon dioxide has proved fatal to laboratory animals. People with heart disease are known to be prone to cardiac arrhythmia due to inhalation of carbon dioxide.[31]

According to an NAS committee report, "the carbon dioxide concentration associated with a given ventilation rate...can be estimated with confidence. For a rate of 9.7 cubic feet per minute [of fresh air] per occupant [passenger], the carbon dioxide concentration would be about 0.15 percent, or 1,500 parts per million. No adverse health effects of carbon dioxide would be noted at this concentration, but the FAA standard for aircraft allows for double this concentration." The latter figure is a concentration of carbon dioxide 12 times higher than that which applies to the general population.[32]

The FAA standard is several decades old and, according to the NAS, "is much higher than standards for other confined environments. The committee recommends that the FAA review its carbon dioxide standard."[33]

Trapped Gas ✈

Low air pressure causes more than just oxygen deficiency, Bertil Werjefelt reminded senators during their aviation safety hearings: "The heart is forced to increase its rate in order to compensate to provide an equal amount of oxygenated blood to the vital areas of the body." Within a low-oxygen airplane cabin, the nitrogen level in the body increases to 20 percent. Since the body cannot burn off nitrogen, it must be released through respiration. This takes place slowly, and in the meantime the body swells with trapped nitrogen gas.[34]

The AMA's Commission on Emergency Medical Services notes that "air or gas trapped in body cavities expands in direct proportion to the decrease in pressure." In an airplane cabin with a simulated altitude of 6,000 to 8,000 feet, the gas would expand about 25 percent (enough to cause a lot of discomfort). Therefore, the AMA advises that individuals "not fly during the congestive stages of an upper respiratory tract disease." The AMA also notes that trapped gas in dental fillings, abscesses, and cavities may cause toothache during ascent, so regular checkups before flying are recommended.

"Commercial air transport is contraindicated in patients with pneumothorax, congenital pulmonary anomalies, known diseases of the bowel, or trapped air in any other area of the body," according to the AMA. Flying should be deferred for fourteen days after urologic or gastrointestinal tract surgery. Flying too soon after eye and tooth surgery can also be painful.

The investigating committee of the NAS has confirmed that changes in cabin air pressure have a direct impact on the dissociation of oxygen from hemoglobin.[35] The resulting lack of adequate oxygen concentration in the blood may be uncomfortable and possibly dangerous for people with chronic lung problems, heart disease, anemia, and sickle-cell disease.

Swelling and Bloating ✈

Since flying can sometimes cause the body to swell with gas, passengers may find it much more comfortable to wear loose-fitting clothes on a plane trip. Some passengers choose to wear jogging suits or other sportswear and change to business attire at their final destination.

A drop in cabin pressure can cause gas expansion in the body, so gastrointestinal bloating is not uncommon during the flight sequence. Eating gassy foods prior to flying is obviously not advisable. If abdominal pain from gas does occur, try to pass the gas rather than hold it in.

Air Pressure and Pregnancy ✈

Pregnant women may undergo painful swelling while flying due to changes in air pressure. In certain circumstances this swelling could add complications to their pregnancy. The AMA's Commission on Emergency Medical Services recommends that flying be discontinued beyond the eighth month of pregnancy due to the threat of miscarriage.[36]

San Diego physician Kenneth Lynn Jones and other members of the Research Committee on Flying's Effect on Reproductive Systems believes women should not fly at all while pregnant.

Policies differ among airlines, but their restrictions are usually to minimize inflight deliveries than to promote the health of the mother or fetus. As of early 1994, British Airways has actually required a doctor's note from women more than 27 weeks pregnant in order for them to fly, Virgin Atlantic sought permission in person from the physician or nurse of women over 32 weeks pregnant, and Lufthansa flatly refused to let women fly after their 34th week of pregnancy. Further, American Airlines required a physician's note on its international flights within 30 days of a baby's due date.

Air Pressure and Scuba Diving ✈

Scuba diving is an enjoyable pastime for many people, but experienced divers know that as water depth and pressure increases, the body traps nitrogen gases in its tissues and joints. When a diver surfaces, these colorless, odorless gases are gradually excreted from body fluids and breath. This is without consequence to the diver if the excretion of gas bubbles is slow and pressure differences are not great. However, if a vacationer dives in the morning and catches an afternoon flight back home, he or she may be in for trouble due to the combined trauma to the body.

Once a plane reaches cruising altitude, its cabin is kept at or below an air pressure comparable to about 8,000 feet above sea level. The expansion of intestinal gas is just one uncomfortable side-effect of pressurization that affects fliers. If there happens to already be additional trapped gas in the tissues, as is the case for those who have been diving within the preceding 24 hours, there is an increased danger of decompression sickness (also known as "the bends"). Symptoms can range from a dull pain in the joints to a more rare and dangerous reaction that causes damage to the nervous system. It is strongly recommended that scuba divers fly no sooner than 12 hours (preferably 24) after a dive.

Author and scuba diver Michael Emmerman, who recorded data on 152 flights, noted that the average elapsed time from takeoff to cruising altitude was 19 minutes, and that after the aircraft reached cruising altitude the average cabin-adjusted altitude was between 5,000 and 6,500 feet. Emmerman believes that "few commercial aircraft actually expose the passenger to an 8,000 foot cabin altitude and negative cabin environmental elements have contributed to cases where divers suffered symptomatic decompression sickness [the bends]." He suggests that "the basis for determining a maximum critical altitude for flying after diving should be reevaluated [i.e., a 5,000-foot assumption is more realistic than 8,000-foot]."[37]

Other Air Pressure Problems ✈

The symptoms of flying-related air pressure changes and hypoxia are varied. They include sleepiness, lightheadedness, dizziness, headaches, swelling of the body, poor night vision, general feelings of lethargy, and a decline in performance. Common behavioral side-effects that can be readily noticed include: fellow passengers yawn and nod off, flight attendants jump up to drink a fast stimulant, and cockpit crew members start ringing for coffee service, doing anything to stay alert.[38]

When commercial air travel first became popular, chewing gum and candy were often passed out to passengers before take-off and landing because the swallowing action helped equalize air pressure in the ears. The ascent and descent of most planes cause pressure changes which affect the middle ear and sinuses. Pressure inside the middle ear must "equalize" to that of the exterior environment. Ascent causes air to flow out of the middle ear and into the throat through the Eustachian tubes. Descent, on the other hand, requires air to flow back into the middle ear. This process may be difficult to achieve without forced swallowing.[39]

If you have allergies or a cold, permanent damage to your ear, nose, and throat can occur if air pressure is not equalized, especially upon descent. Some people have sustained ear and sinus injury so severe that they can never fly again. The pain can be excruciating. (Remedies are offered in the next section.)

During my first year as a flight attendant I was grounded for almost two months after sustaining a hemorrhage behind the eardrum. While on reserve duty, I was ordered by a supervisor to work a flight even though I had a head cold. I endured tremendous pain as tissues expanded in my sinuses and ears, already swollen from the cold. The pain upon descent was almost blinding. I was rushed to a hospital, where doctors advised me not to fly or even ride in an elevator for at least six weeks or until the hemorrhage had dissolved.

How to Reduce Respiratory Injury When You Fly ✈

It would be nice if the nutritional supplements and antioxidants described later in this book were enough to compensate for the lack of fresh oxygen inside aircraft cabins.

While nutrients such as chlorophyll, iodine, iron, beta-carotene, and vitamins A, C, and E can improve the body's use of available oxygen, there really is no substitute for fresh air.

Descending from higher altitude is the most problematic time for those with obstructed air passages, since congested Eustachian tubes require some help equalizing pressure in the middle ear. Using a technique known as the "Valsalva Method" during descent may alleviate pain and reduce the risk of ruptured eardrums. Start by closing your mouth and pinching your nostrils shut, then gently blow air until you hear a popping sound or feel air passing through your ear and sinus passages.

Babies or very young children often have air pressurization problems on flights because their sinuses and ears are anatomically less able to adjust to these changes. Infants and small children should be encouraged to swallow a lot during takeoff and landing, perhaps by offering them a bottle or pacifier. If your baby cries, allow him or her to do so since it helps keep those passages open. If the crying continues beyond a reasonable length of time, however, have the child's ears examined by an ear specialist as soon as possible.

Ozone Hazards ✈

Ozone forms a gaseous layer that surrounds and protects the earth from the intense ultraviolet radiation of the solar system. The ozonosphere ranges from 80,000 feet to 100,000 feet in altitude, just above the 60,000-foot level flown by the SST aircraft (popularly known as the Concorde).

Excessive ozone can be highly toxic, causing pain and tightness in the chest. Occupational Safety and Health Administration guidelines warn that ozone "may cause pulmonary edema [fluid retention in the lungs and heart] at high exposure."[40] Long-term exposure to ozone can be exacerbated by even an aspirin.[41]

The earth's ozone layer has somewhat erratic and can extend in vertical streaks from the ozonosphere downward to all altitude levels. At certain times of the year the ozone concentration tends to be greater in the northern latitudes. Planes flying at 45,000 feet, from the West Coast to Japan or over the polar ice cap to Europe, may encounter especially high levels of ozone on these routes during March, April, and May.

In her Senate aviation subcommittee testimony, Lisa Yates, a flight attendant who chaired Pan American Airlines' health and safety committee, pointed out that many international polar flights routinely soar above 40,000 feet, substantially higher than the standard altitude of 25,000 to 35,000 feet for shorter domestic routes. Flying this high is a cost-saving procedure that allows for lower fuel consumption, though it also exposes passengers and crew to increased concentrations of ozone, not to mention solar and cosmic radiation.

Yates told senators that when Pan Am flight attendants first reported symptoms of what they believed to be ozone poisoning, airline officials dismissed them as "hysterical females." Ironically, during this same period, the company's head physician was collecting data which suggested that flight attendants flying extremely high-altitude routes were indeed developing chronic respiratory problems. The Pan Am health department was closed shortly thereafter, reportedly because of labor-related costs.[42]

Atmospheric ozone enters aircraft via intake vents on a plane's air packs and tends to remain in the cabin until exhausted through outflow valves (which are frequently clogged). Foresight on the part of the SST's designers included a means for destroying ozone by high engine heat levels before outside air is introduced into the plane's cabin. In the past, some airlines have also installed catalytic converters or charcoal filters to reduce ozone contamination. They reportedly proved ineffective, however, and are no longer used on U.S. commercial aircraft.

The FAA and even some airlines have suggested that flight attendants monitor the cabin air by means of their own physical discomfort, requesting that cockpit crews turn on all air packs when ozone contamination seems to have become excessive. Unfortunately, this can lead to a conflict if the crews have been told to conserve fuel by keeping a pack turned off whenever possible.

The Aviation Consumer Action Project has found that passengers are unwittingly monitoring ozone levels by their physical reactions, too. This takes the form of shallow breathing, gasping for air, and bulging eyes. Passengers have actually been observed sitting with pillowcases over their heads because of their extreme discomfort. Ozone is very irritating to the lungs but, unfortunately, pillowcases will not filter it from the air.

During aviation subcommittee hearings on cabin air quality, Senator Nancy Kassebaum (R-KS) asked Craig Beard, the FAA's Air Worthiness Administrator, whether his agency consistently monitored ozone levels in commercial airliners. "No, Senator," Beard replied. "We do not monitor them during the operation of the aircraft except in the ozone area [ozonosphere]. . . . It is more of a subjective evaluation."[43] This is only one of many on-the-record illustrations of the FAA's indifferent attitude toward the health hazards affecting today's flying public.

While the FAA and the airlines they regulate choose to ignore the ozone problem, evidence of its destructive nature continues to mount. Researchers have discovered that the compound mimics the effects of ionizing radiation and may form a destructive chain reaction that can cause chromosome and cellular damage, poison the body, and change mental functions.[44]

The effect of excess ozone on the body can even become life threatening. A retired international flight attendant interviewed on the "CBS Morning News" had been given three electrocardiograms within one year for symptoms that suggested a heart problem, although those results proved negative. The attendant experienced tightness and pain in the chest during flight, along with headaches and dizziness. These are also symptoms of excessive ozone consumption. Since her discomfort occurred only during flight, she and Dr. David Hawkins of the Natural Resources Defense Council realized ozone poisoning was the cause. When the woman stopped flying, her problems disappeared.

Hundreds of symptoms reported by flight attendants have been attributed to ozone poisoning. These include blurred vision, eye irritation, headaches, edema, disorientation, and spitting up blood. Many flight attendants have sought private medical assistance and their physicians have concurred that these particular health problems "appear to be work related. Symptoms also include coughing, upper airway irritation, a tickle in the throat, chest discomfort, substernal pain or soreness, difficulty or pain in taking a breath, shortness of breath, wheezing and nasal congestion."[45]

C.E. Melton, an official of the FAA's Civil Aeromedical

Institute, has cited research stating that cabin ozone concentrations of over 1.0 parts per million (ppm) by volume have been found in airline cabins. Melton feels that even "brief exposure" to this level may be more likely to cause ozone sickness than a sustained exposure to 0.30 ppm. His review also indicates that people with pulmonary diseases may be more susceptible to ozone poisoning, and high levels of the harmful substance may promote the spread of streptococcal infection.

Melton feels there is some question as to whether people can actually adapt to ozone exposure, although specific studies with animals suggest that a tolerance to brief ozone exposures can develop rapidly.[46] The continuous experimental exposure of mice to high levels of ozone did more damage than intermittent exposure at the same levels, eventually leading to chronic diseases.[47]

Federal Air Regulations state that "the airplane cabin ozone concentration during flight must be shown not to exceed .25 ppm (by volume) sea level equivalent, at any time above flight level 320 (32,000 feet at standard atmosphere); or .01 ppm during any three-hour interval above flight level 270 (27,000 feet)."[48]

The NAS 1986 Report noted the following: "Ozone has been measured at concentrations above 0.8 parts per million by volume (ppmv) in the cabin during flights above the tropopause [36,089 feet] and during periods in which there is increased vertical air exchange between the stratosphere [from the tropopause to 265,000 feet] and the troposphere [sea level to tropopause]. This relatively high concentration can be reduced if ozone control equipment has been installed and is operating or if altitude and route limitations are imposed. In comparison with the observed ozone concentration of 0.8 ppmv, compliance with existing standards would limit ozone concentration to a maximum of 0.25 ppmv at equivalent sea-level pressure. Standards also limit the time-weighted average ozone concentration for any flight segment of over four hours to 0.1 ppmv."

An effective means for alerting pilots about existing areas of high ozone concentration is necessary so that flight altitudes can be altered. However, ozone pockets behave so unpredictably that by the time the clearance for the newly requested altitude is received, that altitude level may also be saturated with ozone. A change in latitude as well as altitude may be needed to avoid high ozone areas.

Although the NAS committee could find no documentation of the effectiveness of the various methods being used by the airlines to control ozone, it suggested that the FAA carry out a carefully designed program to ensure that cabin ozone concentrations comply with existing regulations and to study ozone's effects. Researchers found that a significant increase in the number of mild asthma attacks occurred among passengers when peak ozone concentrations exceeded 0.25 ppm.[49]

The NAS committee also pointed out that since exposure to ozone is regulated, the degree of compliance should be determined by representative monitoring and analysis of the ozone concentrations, taking into account various aircraft types, routes and other factors. It recommended that studies be conducted to determine if ozone has any significant effects on the hypoxia already induced by cabin pressurization to the equivalent of an 8,000 feet altitude.[50]

Federal Air Regulations state that airplanes cannot be operated at an altitude or with ventilation equipment that would result in hazardous cabin ozone concentrations, but ozone detectors are not standard equipment on commercial airliners and ozone predictions are only given to pilots when they ask for them.[51]

Negative and Positive Ions   ✈

Some of the same environmental factors that produce ozone also create ions. Ions are atoms that become electrically charged through the loss or gain of one or more electrons. When an atom loses an electron it becomes positively charged, and when it gains an electron it becomes negatively charged.[52] Negative ions (the "good guys") are formed naturally by lightning, waterfalls, fountains, showers, and ocean waves. Positive ions (the "bad guys") are formed by hot dry winds, auto exhaust and other pollutants, as well as some synthetic fabrics, air conditioners, heaters, and electrical fields. Ions are electrically charged by radiation from the sun and background radiation from the earth.

Airplane cockpits are equipped with radar, electronic devices, and computer systems which produce positive ions. The

aircraft cabin has fluorescent lights and most galleys have microwave ovens, both of which generate positive ions.

The amount of ions in the air and the nature of their charges
have important effects on people: negative ions engender a sense
of well-being, while positive ions tend to make one feel anxious
or depressed. This is why you may feel refreshed after a rain-
storm or grumpy and irritable when it is windy. Some people are
more sensitive than others to the ill effects of positive ions, but
most people seem to like the impact of negative ions.[53] Even
plants grow better in negatively ionized air.

Breathing ion-depleted, positive-charged air (such as that
found in airplane cabins) often leads to discomfort, a lack of energy, mental fatigue, and a loss of efficiency. Ions seem to affect
respiratory infections: negative ions appear to increase resistance
to influenza while positive ions, like ozone, tend to lower one's
resistance. Dr. Albert Krueger, a professor emeritus of bacteri-
ology at the University of California-Berkeley, has reported
successful use of negative ions to treat burn patients, people with
psychoneurotic or anxiety syndromes, and stressed workers in
crowded offices.[54]

Blood Clots ✈

The Air Transportation Commission on Emergency Medical Services has noted that sitting in an airplane for an extended period
of time may result in some pooling of blood in the legs and feet.
This condition may pose a problem, the commission concluded,
"in patients with cardiac insufficiency or preexisting thrombotic
or venous disease with danger of pulmonary embolism [blood
clotting in the lungs]."[55]

British physician Dr. John M. Cruickshank and his two colleagues have observed a link between long flights and an increased incidence of blood clots (thromboses). They believe that
the aircraft environment in coach and prolonged periods of sitting
contribute to what they have termed "economy class syndrome."

Michael N. Emmerman, who has written a book on the
health risks of flying, believes that the lack of humidity in the
cabin environment leads to dehydration, which in turn can cause
the blood to thicken or sludge, risking additional stress on the

circulatory system.[56]

Simple Inflight Leg Exercises ✈

In order to prevent leg aches and sluggish blood circulation in the legs, isometric leg exercises can be done even while seated. Contract the calf muscles by rhythmically tensing the muscles and counting to five, then relaxing them for another five counts. This helps drain the legs of stale blood which has lost much of its life-sustaining oxygen. Repeat this series of contraction and release about ten times to get the blood flowing normally again.

The entire leg can be flexed as well. Imagine you are lifting a very heavy object using your legs as the primary power. All the muscles in the legs should contract tightly while you slowly count to five. Do ten sets of this tensing and relaxing exercise.

Simply lifting your heels and dropping them quickly is another easy exercise your can do to improve leg circulation. This action contracts and relaxes the calf muscles automatically.

Continue to do these exercises periodically throughout your flight. They help relieve leg fatigue and improve circulation while decreasing the probability of developing blood clots and phlebitis (inflammation of the blood vessel membrane) in the legs.[57]

Flying and Your Heart ✈

One group of individuals who are particularly vulnerable to the vagaries of contemporary air travel are those with a susceptibility to heart failure. In their testimony before the Senate's aviation subcommittee, Aviation Safety and Health Association founding director Bertil Werjefelt and former Citizen Health Research Group official Dr. Eve Bargmann revealed that, "on a percentile basis, six or seven of every one hundred travelers with a recent heart trauma die within three or four days of [air] travel. In 1980 and 1981 there were no air carrier accidents, yet in each of those years an estimated one hundred persons died when they were stricken by heart attacks, severe allergic reactions, diabetic comas, seizures, choking and other in flight emergencies."[58]

Werjefelt called for further research on cabin air quality since carbon monoxide "is known to displace the oxygen-carrying capacity of a person's blood. This decreased capacity for transmission of oxygen may contribute to inflight and postflight death of patients with ischemic heart disease."[59] Those who have heart-related health conditions should limit air travel.

Doctors' Advice ✈

People do not always consult doctors before flying, so the National Academy of Sciences strongly recommends that physicians do a better job of alerting their patients about the health risks involved in air travel. If your doctor has not given you medical advice and you suspect that conditions such as air quality and pressure changes will adversely affect you, don't hesitate to ask the flight attendant for an oxygen bottle or other special assistance. It is better to be safe than seriously ill or even dead.[60]

Flying and Preexisting Health Conditions ✈

Those who have had recent eye surgery, acute sinusitis, or ear infection (acute otitis media) may experience potentially serious health problems as a result of flying, according to the AMA. Patients who must fly during the congestive stage of an upper respiratory infection should use local or oral decongestants. Descent from altitude can be most problematic with clogged Eustachian tubes as they don't open properly to equalize ear pressure. (See previous suggestions on how to best deal with this condition.)

Passengers who have had abdominal surgery within two weeks of a flight run higher health risks when flying, as do those suffering acute diverticulitis, ulcerative colitis, acute esophageal varices, or acute gastroenteritis. Individuals with epilepsy (unless it is controlled medically and simulated cabin altitude is never greater than 8,000 feet) may suffer increased symptoms when flying. Greater risks also confront those with recent skull fractures, brain tumors, or a history of violent or unpredictable behavior. Caution is advised if one has anemia (a hemoglobin concentration of less than 8.5 g/dL or a red-cell count below three million/mm^3 in adults), sickle-cell disease (unless cruising altitude does not exceed 22,500 feet), or hemophilia.[69]

Chapter 3

AIRBORNE BACTERIA, VIRUSES, AND DISEASE

Most of us have had the unfortunate experience of suffering from a cold or flu a few days after an airplane trip. But few people make a connection between the onset of their sickness and cabin air. Evidence suggests that the inside of a typical commercial airliner is an amazingly fertile breeding ground for the bacteria and viruses that carry infectious illnesses. Fortunately, there are steps you can take to reduce your airborne susceptibility to disease.

Dr. Elliot C. Dick, a physician, professor of preventative medicine, and leading authority on respiratory virus research, has speculated that aircraft "may be the way we seed much of the country with some of our influenza viruses. Influenza kills people, particularly if they already have compromised pulmonary or cardiovascular systems. Infectious particles extruded during coughing, sneezing, and talking are usually captured in the upper respiratory tract. Efficient aircraft ventilation could significantly modify the dissemination of infection by large particles."[1]

Put simply, Dr. Dick believes better air filtering systems on planes would make a big difference in reducing the spread of infectious diseases. His conclusion makes perfect sense if you think about some of the things we are forced to breathe in the closed environment of an airplane cabin: perspiration, dander, perfume, and the host of microorganisms living in and on our human bodies. All of these, in addition to fungi and molds, are present in an aircraft because they are not removed by filters in the ventilation systems and there is insufficient fresh air ventilation to combat their growth.

The seriousness of disease distribution on airplanes was demonstrated by Dr. Dick in his capacity as head of the University of Wisconsin's Respiratory Virus Research Laboratory. In tests conducted within the cabin of a Boeing 727 en route from Chicago to Washington, Dr. Dick detected 127 colonies of infectious organisms transmitted by human beings. The microorganisms accumulated on three petri dishes set out 40 minutes prior to takeoff (during a common traffic delay) and on another four dishes opened during the 70-minute flight. The most significant results appeared on plates placed on passenger seats: 117 colonies were present on the petri dish opened before takeoff and 125 on the dish opened during flight. Staphylococcus was the most common organism detected, along with other bacteria and molds.

Michael N. Emmerman, administrator for the National Association for Search and Rescue, found bacterial colony counts as high as 256 per petri dish during his own inflight tests. By way of comparison, dishes opened in restaurants showed no more than fourteen colonies over the same time span.[2]

Unsterilized Sweat and Breath   ✈

Bertil Werjefelt, founding director of the Aviation Safety and Health Association, told the Senate's aviation subcommittee that "95 percent of the moisture in the air on board an aircraft is unsterilized sweat and breath. It is virtually impossible to encounter circumstances, other than our aircraft, where this occurs."

"With the recent advent of the fuel crisis," Werjefelt continued, "airlines have reduced the input of fresh air to between five and seven cfpm [cubic feet per minute per person] for fuel conservation measures. By doing so, the relative humidity rises to a high of approximately 20 percent (almost all of it perspiration and expiration). In order that passengers have a feeling of reasonable ventilation, approximately 70 percent of the used air is recirculated. The cockpit crew is, by a separate ventilation system, provided essentially 100 percent fresh air."[3]

The same topic was discussed during a 1985 subcommittee hearing by witness Paul Halfpenny, vice chairman of the National Research Council's Committee on Cabin Air Quality. Chairman Daniel Inouye interrupted Halfpenny to ask: "You mean I get my humidity by taking in your breath and perspiration?" "And vice versa," Halfpenny responded. "Yes, sir."[4]

Cabin Conditions Perfect for Disease   ✈

Oxygen and humidity are greatly reduced in a pressurized cabin environment, thus providing the perfect habitat for growth of airborne bacteria. "At 30,000 feet or any other cruise altitude," Paul Halfpenny informed the Senate during his testimony, "the absolute humidity is down in the [range of] one grain per pound. That is extremely dry, essentially zero."

During the questioning, Senator Inouye asked Elliot Dick if the respiratory virus researcher was convinced "that the potential for severe medical problems does exist" in the cabin environment. "I certainly am," Dr. Dick replied, without hesitation, "Most epidemiologists tracing chains of transmission generally separate the route [of infection] into two broad categories, contact and airborne. . . . Contact transmission suggests direct movement of the causative microbe from person to person by actual physical contact, e.g., shaking hands, or by sequential handling of an inanimate object such as the handle of a flush toilet. Contact transmission is probably most important in those upper respiratory infections characterized chiefly by a runny nose [Rhinorrhea]. Infectious particles extruded during coughing remain airborne for an extended time and can penetrate deep within the lung of the recipient. Large particles can fall from the air within a few feet and within a few minutes. When inhaled, these particles are usually captured in the upper respiratory tract."

Although the cabin air is very arid, Dr. Dick expressed concern about "bacteria and fungi which are nearly always growing at the moist air exits or in the water storage areas [of airplanes].

This microbial proliferation may be very important, as one of the water-loving organisms, Legionella, causes a severe [and potentially deadly] pneumonia, Legionnaire's Disease."

Fungi and actinomycetes can tolerate both wet and dry surfaces or cycles and temperature extremes, all of which are present in the aircraft environment. A report from a flight attendant flying throughout the Pacific and the Orient out of Honolulu stated that crew members are being treated for rare tropical diseases that the doctor believes inhabit their aircraft's air vents.[5]

Dr. Dick cited a documented case of an airborne illness in an aircraft that reached epidemic proportions: "It was in a 737—taking off from Homer, Alaska, and bound for Kodiak—whose port engine failed on takeoff. On that plane of fifty-three passengers was a woman who was acutely ill with influenza [laboratory diagnosed]. She spread her virus to 72 percent of the other individuals on that plane—probably during the time the aircraft was delayed on the ground. Four people were hospitalized. It is extraordinarily fortunate that nobody died, because influenza kills people. It is a dangerous virus, particularly for anybody with a compromised pulmonary or cardiovascular system."

Senator Inouye asked Dr. Dick if he was suggesting that an infectious incident like this could happen in other circumstances and not be detected. "It is extremely likely that it has occurred many times," said the doctor, arguing that such an outbreak could be easily prevented with better oversight of cabin air quality. "In fact, disinfection of the air we breathe is one of the few measures we have to control respiratory illnesses."[6]

Low-Humidity Problems   ✈

Airborne bacteria thrive in arid environments, but lack of moisture can cause health problems as well. The brain, like the rest of the body, is subject to dehydration, which in turn may lead to disorganized thinking. Symptoms of dehydration include severe thirst, eye irritation and blurred vision, respiratory problems, impacted colon, risk of kidney stones, sodium-potassium metabolism disturbance, nausea, vertigo, blocked sinuses and eardrums, and dry mucous membranes that are less resistant to infection.

Chronic exposure to the low humidity on airplanes may

make fliers more susceptible to any of these conditions and possibly others.[7] One study, for example, found that urinary calculosis (stone formation) was common to flight personnel and "possibly attributable to low humidity."[8]

The FAA claims that there is no real need for additional moisture inside commercial airliners. In a revealing comment, Dr. Don Jordon, Deputy Federal Air Surgeon for the FAA, told the Senate's aviation subcommittee that he saw "humidity principally as a matter of comfort, not a matter of health." The physician insisted that "to require significant amounts of humidity in the aircraft is probably not practical, nor indicated from a medical point of view. . . . No one could be more allergic than I," Jordan continued, "yet I fly quite a bit. I do not notice any deleterious effects from flying on my nasal or mucous membranes."

In its official comments on the humidity issue, the FAA has noted that moisture inside houses and cars during the winter often fall as low as 5 or 6 percent and that this poses "no significant health problem." However, winters in chilly climates are also commonly known as cold and flu seasons, and influenza is a deadly disease for many people every year.

Senator Inouye's response to Dr. Jordan's comment was blunt. "I am certain the good doctor is well aware that the most common reason for doctor visitations in the United States is respiratory problems. I travel enough to know that usually 50 percent of the time there is someone around me with some respiratory problem, and I can imagine the discomfort and the physical problems that may be encountered by that passenger. Whenever you go into a hospital with some respiratory problem, they shove humidity by the pound upon you, and for any doctor to say that humidification is not necessary is just beyond me. I think he had better go back to his books again and check with those doctors who deal with respiratory problems."[9]

An FAA official conceded during the Senate hearings that on flights longer than three hours, low humidity becomes a problem for some passengers, and that people with respiratory disorders experience discomfort at humidity levels lower than 30 percent.

Relative humidity is a combination of moisture and heat. Whatever the humidity on the ground, it is decreased at higher altitudes by the cooler temperatures found there.[10] The FAA contends that maintaining cabin humidity levels of over 30 percent poses certain weight and design problems for commercial carriers. The water they carry needs to be distilled because dissolved minerals may otherwise clog or corrode aircraft equipment. When moisture comes into contact with cold surfaces, it condenses, posing a potential problem inside the cabin if temperatures are not kept high enough. Keeping the interior cool and dry is one problem, but a cold and clammy environment would likely make passengers even more uncomfortable.

Bertil Werjefelt who testified that domestic airlines could easily humidify their cabins at levels of 20 to 25 percent. British Airways has been doing this for the past twenty years on its longer flights, Werjefelt pointed out, and the added weight of water costs perhaps an additional fifty cents per passenger.

Humidity Level Recommendations ✈

The National Academy of Sciences (NAS) concluded that forced-air ventilation was warranted due to the potential risk of spreading infectious disease in aircraft sitting on the ground. "We recommend that no aircraft with passengers on board remain on the ground without operational forced ventilation for longer than one-half hour," the NAS aviation research committee said. "Open doors are not adequate ventilation sources in this situation. If this cannot be done, the passengers should be returned to the terminal." The report went on to say that "if the risk of infection is to be minimized, the amount of outside air supplied to each passenger during flight should be maximized, because outside air at cruise altitude is essentially clean."[11]

Flight crews report that some airlines bypass the procedure by detaching from the gate to wait for taxi clearance.

Pets Need Humidity (and Care), Too ✈

For those who ship animals in the cargo area, remember that they get thirsty, too. Provide a spill-proof water container in their carriers, because turbulence, flight transfers, delays, cancellations, and misplaced baggage might mean that they will be sitting for hours, sometimes days, without food and water. Until 1991, animals were grounded once the outdoor temperature hit 85 degrees unless the carrier provided a cooler environment, but airlines may now transport any animal unless it seems in distress.

In a 1992 letter to *Condé Nast Traveler* magazine, passenger Ethel E. De Loach recalled the words of a pilot who told her: "If you love your pet, leave it at home." The penalty of fining airlines guilty of animal neglect, De Loach concluded, "would not console me for ill treatment of my pet." (U.S. airlines were fined over $50,000 in 1992 for violating animal safety codes.)

Contact the airline in advance to check regulations and services. Most carriers require pets be at least eight weeks old and weaned at least five days prior to flying. Current health and rabies vaccination certificates are likely to be required. Whenever possible, shipping your pet by a direct flight is recommended.

Disease Transmission ✈

A Honolulu newspaper once reported that a traveler on a flight to Hawaii from the East Coast contracted chicken pox and subsequently passed the disease to his wife. While usually benign in children, this disease can be quite severe in adults.

I remember working a particular flight when, just before landing, a fellow crew member raced forward and told me there was a passenger in her section who was vomiting blood. By the time the man could be reached, the three seats in front of him, those immediately adjacent, and the surrounding floor were covered with clotted blood, from an internal bleeding ulcer. After landing, the man was taken by ambulance to a nearby hospital. The airline's station manager, however, did not want to take the time involved with contacting an outside cleaning crew and asked the cabin and ground crew to clean the area. Fresh coffee grounds were spread over the area to partially cover the odor and the plane took off with a full load. New passengers actually sat in those same seats, and food was served after cleanup. At each stop the crew was advised that the upholstery and carpeting would be changed. They were not. I learned subsequently that the plane flew three more days without being cleaned properly.

Another incident occurred when a woman from a developing country, unaware of onboard toilets, stood in the aisle and defecated under her floor-length skirt. The attendant froze the feces with a fire extinguisher and immediately removed it, but the release of bacteria into the cabin had already taken place.

Confronted with countless daily chances of infection, wouldn't it make sense to check occasionally among flight personnel for the presence of staph and other infectious microorganisms, as is standard procedure for hospital personnel?[12]

It should be noted that The American Society of Travel Agents has commended British Airways and Swissair for their cleanup efforts, which range from thorough cabin disinfection to recycling and even ozone reduction.

Other Suspected Cases of Infection ✈

In early 1992, seventy-six passengers on an Aerolineas Argentinas plane traveling from Buenos Aires to San Francisco (via Lima) contracted cholera after eating meals aboard the aircraft. The organism that causes the illness thrives in water and is passed through careless food preparation. An investigation pinpointed a thirteen-ingredient seafood salad as the source of the contamination, and several airlines serving Latin America subsequently stopped serving fresh vegetable, fruit, and seafood items.

Dr. Charles Erickson, a professor of infectious diseases at the University of Texas-Houston Medical School, recommends covering yourself with a nose handkerchief when an infected person nearby coughs or sneezes. "I hold my nose until the cloud of droplets passes," says Erickson, who also recommends flu shots if a traveler is older or has heart, lung, or kidney disease.[13]

Flight Crews With Infectious Diseases ✈

Members of flight crews frequently continue working while they have active colds, sinusitis, ear infections, or other ailments. They do so knowing that the congestion associated with colds and similar diseases may be injurious to them under rapid air pressure changes. In part they keep working to avoid harassment and possible dismissal by their employers. Some airlines call in flight crew personnel with as few as three sick claims and accuse them of undependability, in an apparent effort to fire them.[14] Remaining on the job is also a way of avoiding having to get the doctor's excuse necessary to claim sick pay and be released to fly again. Flu and colds are serious enough, but the penicillin-resistant strains of staph infection—the notorious "hospital staph"—inhabit aircraft cabins and their occupants. Staph causes pneumonia and sinusitis, but it can also be responsible for cellulitis, endocarditis, furuncles and carbuncles, impetigo, meningitis, osteomylitis, otitis media, prostratitis, and septicemia.[15] How confident can a passenger be that the flight attendant has not coughed on the food or that he or she has washed his or her hands before serving food, or that the interior of the aircraft has been sterilized?

Cockroaches and Outright Filth ✈

The spread of disease in the aircraft cabin is a danger recognized by the Food and Drug Administration, which stipulates that a plane is to be completely fumigated if any cockroaches are found on board. However, flight crews and ground agents face uncomfortable confrontation with management should there be a request for a flight delay or cancellation in order to fumigate. Cockroaches are most often seen in the toilet areas—frequently located near the galleys—where the insects scavenge food.[16] Salmonella is one of the many dangerous bacteria carried by the cockroach.

A flight attendant with whom I was acquainted telephoned me once with a real horror story. One of the toilets aboard the DC-10 she was working had overflowed into the passenger aisle and galley area after someone tried to flush a dirty diaper.

"There were visible lumps [of human feces] on the galley floor," my friend exclaimed, confiding that she and the other flight attendants were aghast at the prospect of preparing and serving food in such an environment.

While one attendant notified the captain, the other ran off the plane to call the local health department. Upon learning the identity of the airline involved, the health department representative said that nothing could be done. The captain called his superiors, returned sheepishly to the aircraft, and said the mess would be dealt with as best as possible by the cleaning crew, without the carpeting being fully replaced. The wet floor and contamination from the sewage still remained, and this was the environment in which passengers received meals. The aircraft flew for months before finally being grounded to have the toilet lines cleared.

Infectious Cargo ✈

You are strongly advised to wash your hands after carrying your luggage from an airplane because cargo areas often carry animals, whose dander, feces, and urine may carry infectious diseases that can be dispersed through the air or on surfaces. Spiders, contaminated baggage, and laboratory microorganisms can also contaminate the passenger baggage compartment.

An official report presented to Congress by the airline safety and hazard committee of the NAS indicates that "the greatest danger from cargo sources would be associated with pathogenic microorganisms in cultures that are damaged during transit. The infective dose of some pathogens is a single cell. Pathogens can be transported by mail and are allowed in passenger aircraft if properly packaged." Laboratories often ship pathogenic specimens or hand carry them on airliners throughout the world.[17]

AIDS ✈

The secretariat of International Civil Aviation Operations has concluded that screening passengers for Human Immunodeficiency Virus (HIV), the virus that causes AIDS, would be impractical. The head of aviation's international regulatory agency—along with medical experts—does not believe that there is a risk of infection from sharing the same cabin space. The secretariat also does not believe that "the presence of positive serology for HIV should disqualify aviation personnel from their duties unless there is medical evidence to prove otherwise."

Whether or not other passengers might be infected by a person with AIDS is not the central issue. Rather, the HIV-positive passenger should consider that his or her health may be placed at risk due to the cabin's dry air and infectious contents.

Some alert doctors are already advising their AIDS patients not to fly on the grounds that their weakened immune systems cannot easily cope with the compromised environment. Elliot Dick offered the following for consideration:

"Tuberculosis may be a new problem for civilian aircraft passengers. With the advent of AIDS, tuberculosis has made something of a renaissance. Persons infected with the AIDS virus have a depressed immune system, and tuberculosis has become an important pathogen for them. I wonder how often some of these relatively healthy AIDS patients with tuberculosis travel unknown on commercial aircraft. It is well known that tuberculosis is spread almost entirely through the air and can remain alive for extended periods of time. This is an organism which can cause an insidious and lethal infection. The tubercle bacillus is also very resistant to antiseptics." In a 1993 follow-up letter, Dr. Dick reiterated that "tuberculosis could be a severe problem on planes if employees are infected with the AIDS virus. Drug-resistant tuberculosis organisms spread rapidly among persons with AIDS and it is often hard to detect...Both cholera and tuberculosis could be real problems to airline personnel and to passengers."[18]

A flight attendant told me about an AIDS patient who was flying from Honolulu to San Francisco. Although the man started out on the five-hour trip feeling fine, by the time it was nearing its end he was in a coma and running a fever so high that the attendant could feel the heat a foot away from his body. The passenger had to be removed from the aircraft by a paramedic team.

Consideration should be given to recent epidemics of tuberculosis in New York, polio in Holland, cholera in Latin America, as well as such widespread diseases as hepatitis, malaria, and AIDS. With this in mind, the European Community imposed new laws on January 1, 1993, making it a criminal offense for tour operators and travel retailers to fail to inform their customers about health risks and requirements before a journey.[19]

Immigration Flights ✈

The deportation of undocumented aliens from the United States back to their home countries is a matter of concern to international passengers, who may sometimes find themselves either on the same commercial flights used to deport these individuals or on aircraft chartered by the Immigration and Naturalization Service (INS) for this purpose.

Known AIDS patients and others with infectious diseases are isolated by plastic barriers when transported on deportation flights coordinated by the INS. Disposable clothing, linens, and other items are used for the patients' care, although in many cases this is done more for the peace of mind afforded healthy passengers and crew rather than to prevent transmission of the disease.

Despite such precautions, occurrences of various infections are high on these flights. One of the more common highly contagious diseases encountered is "pink eye" or conjunctival infection of the eye. Most common, but less infectious, is tuberculosis. Given the circumstances under which large numbers of passengers are transported each month on these flights, the potential for spreading disease and the difficulties of maintaining a clean aircraft to control the process represents quite a problem. Some INS nurses believe chlorine will kill the AIDS virus; however, other chemicals are now used in order to avoid chlorine's corroding an airplane's metal surfaces, particularly its frame.

The bathrooms and all surface areas are cleaned, or spot-cleaned when necessary, after every INS load. This includes floors, arms of seats, and metal on seat belts. In addition, every four to six weeks or every five hundred passengers the seats are steamed and the entire aircraft is professionally cleaned. Under ordinary circumstances, commercial airlines find it too costly to take a plane out of service long enough to clean this thoroughly.

The INS implements the following cleaning methods on planes it uses to fly deportees:

- Water containers are sanitized after each flight in a one-cup-per-gallon solution of sodium hypochlorite (liquid bleach), as is the ice chest used to transport food.

- Lavatory surfaces and vinyl seat covers are sprayed after each flight with Cidex (generally known as activated dialdehyde solution, containing 2 percent glutaraldehyde).

- Blankets and clothing, unless disposable, are laundered after each use.

- Carpets on which people have vomited or urinated, or where food has been spilled, are first scrubbed with clear water to remove the large particles. Then a solution of tincture of green soap or hexachlorophene is scrubbed into the carpet until a lather forms. The carpet is then scrubbed for five to ten minutes and rinsed. It is steam-cleaned monthly or sooner.[20]

Chapter 4

RADIATION IN FLIGHT

Despite the recommendations of many experts, airplane crew members and passengers are not subject to the same kinds of safety regulations and precautions applied to ground-based radiation workers, even though their work or travel involves exposure to unusually high levels of ionizing radiation. When an airliner is traveling at high altitudes, those aboard are constantly bombarded by naturally occurring radiation from the sun, stars, and other celestial objects—radiation that is filtered out at lower levels of the atmosphere. Research has shown that exposure to high doses of such radiation—which also emanates from medical X-rays, nuclear power plants, radioisotope drugs, and the earth itself—can cause cancer, as well as other diseases and disorders.

Radiation, in varying amounts and of various types, is virtually everywhere. Yet most air travelers and many of those who fly for a living have no knowledge or understanding of the high-altitude radiation risks of flying, safe dosages of radiation, how radiation exposure is measured, or even the different kinds of radiation. Therefore, a brief summary of up-to-date scientific information about radiation and its effects may be helpful.

Radiation exists at all levels in our environment. The element radium is naturally present in the soil, for example, and trace amounts of radioactive materials enter and leave our bodies all the time through the food we eat. Cosmic rays from the sun and the stars have an effect on us as well. We gain some additional exposure to radiation through various medical therapies and diagnostic procedures, such as routine dental and chest X-rays.[1]

Radiation and Altitude ✈

Solar and stellar sources of radiation are of special concern for anyone who flies frequently. In general, these radiation levels vary according to altitude and latitude. The higher one flies and the closer one gets to the poles, the more the radiation exposure.

Dr. Edward T. Bramlitt, a health physicist with the Defense Nuclear Agency, once noted in an address to the Aerospace Medical Association that flight altitudes used by high-flying commercial and corporate jets, as well as the Super Sonic Transport (more commonly known as the SST or Concorde), expose everyone on board to neutrons ranked twenty times more harmful than gamma radiation—which are similar to X-rays but shorter in length. U.S. government monitoring shows an average of about seven major solar flares (radiation bursts) a year, with at least one strong enough to affect the neutron flux at ground level.

Radiation absorbed by body tissues in bone marrow, or by a fetus in the uterus, is expressed in milliSieverts (mSv). Sieverts represent a newer terminology of the dose equivalent biological impact of radiation on exposed human beings.[2] This unit of measurement has replaced the older rem measurement: 1 rem = 0.01 Sv (10 milliSieverts).

In order to give these scientific terms a more human dimension, a person living at sea level in New York is exposed to 0.26 mSv per year, while a person living in Denver at 5,280 feet elevation is exposed to 0.50 mSv per year. The difference in exposure is caused by the shielding effect of the atmosphere at lower altitudes. Cosmic ray exposure is thought to double for every 6,500 feet gained in elevation from sea level.

Exposure to celestial radiation also increases as one moves toward either of the earth's poles. Thus at 70° N latitude (the

Arctic Circle, which passes through northern Canada, Alaska, and Siberia) a person is exposed to roughly four times the radiation experienced at 25°N latitude (the Tropic of Cancer, which encompasses such cities as Mazatlan, Mexico). Within the United States, the cities of Denver and Philadelphia rest on latitude 40°N and split the difference in exposure between the two previous examples. Radiation can also increase rapidly because of occasional solar flares and other geomagnetic events.

Radiation's Impact on Passengers and Crews   ✈

California radiologist Dr. Donald Cusick asserts that "every transcontinental flight is worth at least one chest X-ray" in terms of radiation exposure. Dr. John Gofman, author of *Radiation and Human Health,* believes that the radiation absorbed during a transcontinental flight is even greater than that.

As recently as 1987, the Department of Transportation (DOT) was downplaying the risk of high-altitude radiation exposure to airline crew members. DOT official Donald Engen, in his *Report to Congress on Airline Cabin Air Quality,* concluded that "crew members at risk of exceeding the 500 millirems annual limit [of allowable radiation exposure under federal law] represent only a small percentage of those engaged in the industry."[3]

(According to a front-page report in the February 14, 1990, edition of the *New York Times*, the average American is exposed to 300 millirems a year of naturally occurring radiation and the average nuclear plant worker a total of 650 millirems annually.)

I asked Dr. Bramlitt, an expert on the subject, for information on the radiation risks associated with flying. *(These are personal opinions of Dr. Bramlitt and do not necessarily reflect the views of his employer—the Department of Defense—or the U.S. government)*

Author: Do flight attendants receive a significant radiation dose during high-altitude flying?

Bramlitt: Relatively speaking, yes. Their annual flying doses are comparable to doses received by members of the nation's radiation work force [such as nuclear power plant workers and X-ray technicians].

Author: Should flight attendants be concerned about the radiation doses they receive?

Bramlitt: Most radiobiologists agree that every level of dose carries some risk of harm, and doses should be avoided unless there is a net positive benefit. The Federal Aviation Administration, as the responsible federal agency for safety in air commerce, should require assessments of the dose each flight attendant receives, and offer training and instruction on the consequences of exposure to radiation. Then rational decisions could be made as to whether the benefits received from flying justify the risks.

How Much Exposure Is Too Much? ✈

Alan Stoker, a hydrogeologist with the Los Alamos National Laboratories in New Mexico, compared radiation risks encountered on commercial flights with "Acid Canyon," the place where the nuclear scientists of Los Alamos discharged their treated and untreated liquid radioactive wastes during the 1940s and 1950s. "Spending a day in Acid Canyon would be less of a risk than the amount of radiation passengers on a cross-country airplane trip are exposed to," Stoker commented.

Risks of cancer caused by radiation for cabin crew members and any other frequent flyers are now found to be much greater than had been previously estimated. On February 19, 1990, *The New York Times* reported an estimate of risk that was revised upward from fifty-nine cancer cases in 100,000 to 1,000 in 100,000.[4] This risk factor is in addition to the estimated 22 percent (22,000 out of 100,000 people) of the total population who are expected to die from cancer.

The revised DOT report, which helped to elucidate these statistics, was prepared by Geomet, Inc. of Germantown, Maryland, a company that specializes in indoor air testing. Dr. Wallace Friedberg, a supervisor in the radiobiology department of the FAA's Civil Aeromedical Institute, has produced a virtually identical "risk coefficient" for cancer in his studies of radiation. Friedberg's study and a draft report by Dr. Robert R. McMeekin, the Federal air surgeon, are discussed later in this chapter.

The *New York Times* estimate of 1,000 air carrier crew members contracting cancer within the lifetimes of a population of 100,000 was based on a statistical model of 100,000 cabin crew members or passengers flying round-trip from New York to Seattle, ninety-eight times a year for twenty years. The risk of cancer rises considerably when flying a polar route from Tokyo to New York. Thirty-seven round-trips a year on that route for ten years would lead to 1,200 fatal cancers in 100,000 people, according to the Geomet study. The risk becomes even greater during periods of sunspot activity.[5] ABC-TV's "Good Morning America" reported a three-day exposure warning for North Pole area flights during a radiation storm caused by solar flare activity.

Flight attendants, cockpit crew members, and all frequent fliers have reason to be concerned. The Union of Flight Attendants and the Association of Flight Attendants (AFA) began reporting a series of potential radiation-related health problems—ranging from birth defects to cancer—among their members as early as 1986, when Matthew Finucane, AFA Director of Safety and Health, testified before Congress.[6]

Interestingly, Finucane was responsible for spotting a crucial error made by the DOT when it released the Geomet study. The department originally reported the risk rate of fifty-nine cancer cases in 100,000, rather than the Geomet estimate of 1,000 in 100,000. The mistake was attributed to "human error."

In 1992, the DOT estimated that passengers on 32 nonstop flights within the U.S. would receive a galactic radiation exposure of up to .8 milliSieverts. For a crew member, this translates to an exposure as high as 7.2 milliSieverts a year. Few crew members, however, have seen this study, or a separate 1992 Office of Aviation Medicine report on inflight radiation risks.[7]

Radiation Standards for Passengers and Crews   ✈

The weight of scientific and anecdotal evidence clearly demonstrates the need to establish radiation exposure standards for flight crew members and other frequent fliers.

Bramlitt has cited the standards set for workers in the atomic industry as one kind of precedent. He has also noted a similar difficulty in measuring the effects of radiation experienced by "atomic veterans," the thousands of military men and women who were exposed to large amounts of radiation in the late 1950s and early 1960s.[8] He compared the atomic veterans' past struggle to gain recognition of their purported radiation-related diseases to the present situation confronting flight attendants.

As Bramlitt states, "Monitoring is needed for safety, to forestall litigation, and possibly to avoid the expense of dose reconstruction in the future as was required for service personnel at nuclear weapon test sites whose doses, by the way, averaged less than the expected flight attendant annual dose."[9]

In an issue of the *Aerospace Medical Association Journal,* an article entitled *Occupational Risks of Flying for a Living: Aviation, Space, and Environmental Medicine*, contained a set of statistical norms compiled by Wallace Friedberg and his colleagues that evaluated the occupational risks encountered by people who fly for a living.[10] Friedberg's work has, to some extent, been echoed in the Geomet study reported in *The New York Times* and is virtually identical to a draft copy of Advisory Circular 120-XX signed by air surgeon Robert R. McMeekin.[11]

Both Friedberg and McMeekin, along with Geomet, have used the same table of "Dose Equivalents from Galactic Cosmic Radiation Received on Air Carrier Flights." This table draws on data from thirty-two flights, which includes their highest altitudes, time aloft, block hours (measured from when the aircraft leaves the blocks prior to takeoff to when it reaches the blocks after landing), radiation dosage for that particular flight, and the dosage for 950 block hours on that same route (equivalent to a year's flying time). Not surprisingly, as they used the same investigative data, each of these researchers came to essentially the same conclusions about the potential impact of ionizing radiation on air travelers and crews.[12]

Low Level Cosmic Radiation →

The Nuclear Regulatory Commission and other federal agencies have determined that 500 millirems (mrem) or 5.0 mSv is the limit of allowable radiation an individual should be exposed to without warning. The National Council on Radiation Protection and Measurement (NCRPM), an industry advisory board, made a recommendation to the federal government as far back as 1987 that the maximum allowable dose be reduced to 100 mrem per year.[13] The board determined that work that causes exposure above this revised limit should be governed by rules set up by the Occupational Safety and Health Administration.

An article in *Science* magazine cited a study that concluded that the risks of low levels of penetrating radiation have been underestimated, and the risk for contracting cancer is actually three to four times greater than previously reported in the National Academy of Science's report to Congress. In the article, Arthur C. Upton, chairman of the National Academy of Science's Fifth Committee on Biological Effects of Ionizing Radiation (BEIR-5), said he expected there would be "some response" from regulatory authorities in the form of tighter standards. Warren Sinclair, president of the NCRP, predicted that the "pressure" of BEIR-5 might cause his organization to consider reducing the recommended maximum occupational exposure limit below 500 mrem per year. However, these changes have not been forthcoming.

Some experts feel we cannot discount any evidence of low level radiation risks to human health. Biologist and former University of California professor John W. Gofman commented on the BEIR-5 risk estimates in his November 1990 newsletter for the Committee for Nuclear Responsibility, a non-profit organization Gofman chairs and whose board of directors includes Nobel Prize-winning chemist Linus Pauling and Stanford University biologist Paul Ehrlich.

"Reasonable risk estimates for radiation-induced cancer from nuclear pollution," Gofman wrote, "are six to 30 times higher per rem of dose than the current estimates from such quasi-official radiation committees as BEIR-5 and UNSCEAR-88. Realistic estimates are developed in [my book, *Radiation-Induced Cancer from Low-Dose Exposure: An Independent Analysis*], step by step, using data from the atomic bomb survivors [of World War II]. BEIR and UNSCEAR also rely on the A-bomb survivors—up to a point. Then, in complete defiance of the human evidence, they divide what the evidence shows by two to ten if low doses are slowly received, as from nuclear pollution."

He continued, "My own best estimate, adjusting the A-bomb data for a U.S. population, is a lifetime risk of fatal cancer of 26.6 fatal cancers per 10,000 persons each receiving a dose of one rem to the whole body. This value applies to doses which are spread over time as well as to doses received all at once. . . . By contrast, after the 'two to ten' division, the comparable BEIR-5 risk-values range from 0.86 to 4.28 fatal cancers per 10,000 persons each receiving a one rem dose to the whole body."

Gofman contends in the same newsletter that "proof already exists that there is no safe dose or dose-rate of ionizing radiation. In other words, there is no threshold level below which the risk of radiation-induced cancer disappears. . . . Our analysis leads to the conclusion that low-dose ionizing radiation—including the natural doses—may account for one out of every four cancer deaths. It would be outrageous to increase rather than *decrease* exposures to such a carcinogen. Indeed, since children are much more sensitive than adults to radiation carcinogenesis, it would be a very good idea to reduce childhood exposure to natural background radiation (for instance, from radon, certain building materials, and frequent flying)..."

In *Radiation and Human Health*, one of his four books on the subject, Gofman concludes that among crew members flying 1,000 hours each year, women can expect an increased 1.19 chance per thousand of developing cancer as a result of a year of such work, while men risk an additional 1.49 chance.

"We must always keep in mind that even when something creates a risk which is small *per individual,*" Gofman warns, "it will lead to a sizable number of deaths in a population if *many* individuals are put at that risk. The aggregated effect of many, widespread, small risks—each considered trivial on a personal basis—can be huge." The scientist is convinced that ionizing radiation may turn out to be the most important single carcinogen to which large numbers of humans are exposed.[14]

The studies released by Friedberg, McMeekin, and Geomet conclude that the radiation accumulated per year by a frequent flyer or crew member is nearly double the allowed rate for occupational health.

Captain Kirby A. Van Horn, a Continental Airlines pilot, expressed the problem eloquently in a letter to the FAA: "The average annual radiation that a person gets if living in Texas [at sea level] is approximately 140 millirems per year. So by subtracting this exposure, minus a prorated amount to account for the 950 hours the Air Carrier Crew member is flying and not on the ground (15.18 millirems), from the limit of 500 millirems per year, a result is reached that shows that the Air Carrier Crew member can only receive another 375.18 millirems during the year without exceeding the Nuclear Regulatory Commission limits. Based upon the estimates in Advisory Circular 120-XX of the levels of radiation exposure to Air Carrier Crew members flying at an altitude of 35,000 feet (.06 millirem per hour), this would allow the Air Carrier Crew member to fly at this altitude for 625.3 hours during the year. This compares with the 1,000 hour per year current limitation which, using the above data, yields an annual radiation exposure of 740 millirems."[15]

Captain Van Horn and others have so far spoken only about "average" persons and "average" flying days. People who live at higher altitudes and those who fly more hours than the average expose themselves to greater risks. For example, thousands of air carrier crew members live in Denver and other cities at high elevation. And even the BEIR-5 study concluded that the 500 mrem per year limit should be lowered.

Solar Flares ✈

Our sun occasionally throws off large bursts of radiation. These solar flares (also called "particle events") intensify crew members' chances of developing radiation-induced illnesses. These events, some lasting as long as a week, are sufficiently energetic to cause the radiation field at flight levels to be unusually intense, especially at higher altitudes. The largest event recorded in the past 20 years occurred on March 13, 1989, and displayed 200 to 2,000 times the usual dose of radiation at 39,000 feet—a common cruising elevation for modern jet airliners.

The composition and intensity of cosmic radiation in the atmosphere is not constant, and is more intense near the poles. According to Bramlitt, the increase in altitude from 36,000 to 45,000 feet can effectively double cosmic radiation dosage.

Matthew Finucane, responding to FAA Circular 120-XX, argued that the agency is underestimating the risk undertaken by crew members with respect to radiation.[16] "From 1956 through

1972," he pointed out, "there were four solar particle events during which the dose equivalent rate on polar routes at 41,000 feet probably exceeded 100 microSieverts [10 millirems] per hour. At 40,000 feet, flares can increase the cosmic-radiation dose rate from 0.7 mrem per hour to 200 mrems per hour."

Bramlitt has performed research on solar particle events over a number of years. In a 1989 letter to the Civil Aeromedical Institute's Wallace Friedberg concerning the FAA's draft report on crew member radiation exposure and commenting on the inadequacies of the council's report on the airline cabin environment, Bramlitt presents a list of flares he has documented. He notes that by September 1989, 1,128 hours of actual particle event time had already been experienced during the preceding eight months. This subtotal compares to 602 hours for all of 1988 and 63 hours for 1987. Bramlitt recommends that the FAA report dose estimates at flight levels for each event and mount "a valid and comprehensive radiation monitoring effort at flight levels."

The Need for Epidemiological Research   →

FAA Circular 120-XX has galvanized efforts to classify flying as a hazardous occupation that needs the same kind of radiation monitoring given to those classified officially as atomic workers. Although he has had only limited success in his campaign to get the agency to take more responsible action concerning the special health risks facing airline employees, Bramlitt gives the agency credit for making three critical points in Circular 120-XX:

- Crew member radiation regulations are necessary.
- Crew exposures must be measured accurately.
- Crew members must have access to a professional radiation safety council.

Dr. Robert J. Barish is one of several physicians who has spoken forcefully on the risks taken by crew members. In a letter to the FAA, he urged the agency to "be more forthright in clarifying this [radiation safety] issue and in unequivocally and explicitly presenting the fact that flight crew members are in the mainstream of radiation workers in this country. Their average exposures put them into the ranks of the most exposed individuals for whom the EPA has data.... All air crew members, now and in the future, must be given enough information to enable them to make appropriate personal decisions about their exposures, and to decide if and when the risks might become unacceptable. This is particularly true for pregnant flight attendants or pilots."

Barish concluded that people who have this kind of exposure "deserve the opportunity to decide in real time whether to get on a flight during a large particle event."[17]

Richard B. Stone, executive chairman of aeromedical resources for the Air Line Pilots Association (ALPA), responded by letter to Circular 120-XX and bemoaned the fact that no effort was underway to collect epidemiological evidence to demonstrate the connection between radiation exposure cancer rates.[18]

Stone asked the central questions underlying this chapter: "Do we know whether the incidence or prevalence of leukemia or cancers, for example, is higher in aircrews than for the normal population? Or do we know if any infants of female aircrew members have been born with birth defects attributable to exposure of their mothers to cosmic radiation? . . . Why do we not have epidemiological studies to support action?"

Stone concedes that "the design of such an epidemiological study presents unusual and complicated features, [but] the results would be of significant benefit to aircrew members."

In putting off action until a 1993 proposed FAA rulemaking on radiation, the government and commercial airlines are in danger of creating a legal class of workers that is being exposed to a major health hazard. Flight attendants and other crew members might be compared to the thousands of women who were injured by the Dalkon Shield, a defective intrauterine birth control device, or to the descendants of women who took DES, an experimental drug that harmed themselves and their children.

The Supersonic Example ✈

Monitoring procedures followed on the SST may provide some guidance here, although there is still no requirement that any flight (SST or other) be delayed or forced to descend to a lower altitude to minimize the effect of a solar flare. When the SST became operational in the late 1960s it was recognized that because it was flying at altitudes around 60,000 feet, passengers and crew would be exposed to levels of radiation eight times greater than flights at conventional subsonic altitudes.[19] Consequently, a dosimeter was installed on the aircraft that registered three levels of radiation both on an instantaneous and a cumulative basis.

Curiously, the SST records have been neither published nor publicly analyzed, and the FAA committee which studied SST radiation has been disbanded. Therefore, we do not know if flying the SST has been proven hazardous to its crews or passengers. Still, the practice of recording absorbed radiation on the SST established a precedent for monitoring commercial flights.

Reproductive Disorders and Radiation Exposure ✈

For years, the job-related health problems of unionized flight attendants have been duly noted by their unions and physicians. These workers report greater difficulty in conceiving children, more frequent miscarriages, more stillbirths, and infants born with more physical defects than the rest of the population. They also suffer from fibrous tumors, disturbed menstrual cycles, increased cases of constant nausea, instances of abnormal hair loss, and above normal rates of cancer of the uterus and prostate.

For pregnant flight attendants who fly overtime, there is added danger even though the extra hours may be economically necessary. Although some physicians routinely advise pregnant women against exposure to X-rays and to flying, pregnant flight attendants may be forced to expose their unborn children to the dangers of flight for as much as 15 percent of the child's prenatal life.[20] As University of California pediatrician Kenneth Lyon Jones pointed out, "the womb is not a privileged site."

Gary Ferris, FAA designated senior medical examiner and aviation preventive medicine consultant, stated at an Aerospace Medical Association meeting that insurance records revealed 75 percent of the flight attendants at Continental and Western (now Delta) Airlines reported having miscarried at least once. Studies have shown that all types of childhood cancer and leukemia are doubled by even extremely small doses of radiation.

In one of many stories of personal suffering related by flight attendants who have experienced birth trauma, a Denver-based woman described how she delivered her whole uterus along with her child. Her obstetrician noted that he had observed this phenomenon several times among flight attendants he had treated. In a paper published in 1983 by the Radiation Sciences Division of the U.S. Air Force School of Aerospace Medicine, Dr. David Wood and his colleagues reported "a positive correlation between endometriosis [a disease of the female reproductive system] and radiation exposure." The team worked with a group of rhesus monkeys that had been given a single total body exposure to protons: studies found the monkeys developed illnesses within seven years. The abstract of their article asserts that "the doses and energies of the radiation received were within the range that could be received by an air crew member in near-earth orbit during a random solar flare event."

Wood and his colleagues pointed out that "since spontaneous cases of endometriosis generally occur in older females near the end of their reproductive period, it has been suggested that the radiation effect is an acceleration of the normal aging process." Another study by H.M. McClure suggested that "radiation may alter the immunological response of the host, promoting extrauterine location [displacement of the uterus] and proliferation of endometrial tissue."[21]

Risks to the Unborn ✈

Legitimate concern exists about the risk of birth defects in unborn children resulting from inflight radiation. According to published research, for every 100,000 pregnant women receiving a weekly dose of .05 milliSievert (equivalent to a coast-to-coast round-trip) over the first seven months of their pregnancy, eight miscarriages and thirty-nine children born with birth defects are expected.[22]

John W. Gofman, founder of the Biomedical Research Division of the Livermore National Laboratory, has noted that followup studies on victims of the Hiroshima/Nagasaki bombings of 1945 and the Chernobyl nuclear disaster of 1986 have shown that the exposure of pregnant women and infants to high radiation levels yielded various forms of cancer, birth defects, and mental retardation.[23] He has been disturbed particularly by an increased incidence of thyroid cancer among small children in and around Chernobyl. "Within only five years after the accident," Gofman wrote in a 1992 Committee for Nuclear Responsibility report, "the rate of this cancer has risen to levels far above normal. For years, the radiation community has denied that solid cancers (thyroid, breast, lung, etc.) will occur this early after irradiation. . . . We are sad for humanity and the Chernobyl children that no minimum latent period exists."

In September 1992, the *Los Angeles Times* reported that as many as 71 percent of children born each month during the previous three years in the Siberian city of Talmenka showed symptoms of jaundice and congenital defects in their nervous systems or organs. One prominent Moscow researcher called the babies "nuclear mutants," suggesting their ailments are directly related to radiation exposure linked to the Chernobyl accident, weapons testing, and nearby dumping of radioactive waste.

The study by Friedberg of the FAA cites the same evidence of radiation risk to the fetus as does the definitive 1989 FAA report (Circular 120-XX) on the subject. The latter document makes no attempt to be comprehensive on this topic and, in fact, the discussion is relegated to the appendix. The FAA postulates that a female flying 290 flights between Minneapolis and New York is exposed to an estimated 0.011 mSv per flight.

The agency's report states that during the first week after conception, "before the embryo becomes implanted in the wall of the uterus, the principal danger from radiation exposure is death *in utero*. . . . During the third through the eighth week of pregnancy the principal health concern from radiation exposure is structural abnormalities. During the ninth through the twenty-sixth week of pregnancy the principal concern from radiation exposure is severe mental retardation." From the ninth week through the sixteenth week the risk coefficient is 40 in 100,000, while from the seventeenth week through the twenty-sixth week the risk coefficient is 10 in 100,000.

"A child irradiated *in utero* is at risk of developing childhood cancer," the report concluded. "In general, where more than one of several events may occur together, as in the present case, a simple summation of individual risks will overestimate the risk that at least one of the events will occur; however, for the number and magnitude of the risks under consideration the bias is insignificant."[24]

Gofman's analysis of the Atomic Bomb Survivor Group, however, found that Japanese children irradiated in utero (at the eighth-to-fifteenth weeks of pregnancy) by as little as four rads were nearly six times as likely to be mentally retarded as the general, non-irradiated population.

Dr. Richard L. Master, an aeromedical advisor to the ALPA, suggests flight attendants go on maternity leave as soon as they learn of their pregnancy. Health physicist Bramlitt recommends that women take leave at the time they plan to conceive.

Protecting Yourself from Radiation   ✈

Obviously, you can reduce your exposure to radiation by not flying at all, or by at least flying less. Unfortunately, these options are not possible for most air carrier crew members or others whose livelihoods require they travel long distances.

Excess radiation is a silent enemy. As demonstrated in this chapter, there exists enough accumulated medical data to show that chronic long-term exposure to low doses of radiation alters survival rates and disease incidence statistics in an exposed population. Effects of short exposure high-dosage radiation—such as that accompanying the bombing of Nagasaki and Hiroshima—manifest themselves within days, hours, or even minutes. Skin burns, nausea, and vomiting may occur, along with anemia and weakness. Death can occur within one-to-two weeks.

In contrast, long-term exposure to lower dose radiation has few, if any, short-term biological effects, although these generally can be overlooked or confused with routine illness. For instance, the effects on cellular chromosomes demonstrate genetic birth defects in children only with subsequent reproduction. There is also a statistically significant increase in defects in those exposed populations. Over a period of prolonged exposure, low-level radiation can result in some very serious illnesses.

Radiation exposure may also cause an increase in free radical formation in tissues and cells. Free radicals are molecules that have become activated and are toxic to cell membranes. Recent research shows that free radical production in the body is directly related to the onset of many chronic diseases, such as

atherosclerotic heart disease, cancer, and arthritis. These molecules are produced naturally by the body during metabolic reactions, but their production is increased by environmental toxins,
toxic metals, and saturated dietary fats.

Nutritional Guidelines for Neutralizing Radiation ✈

Antioxidants tend to diminish the effects of free radical (or oxidant) damage to tissues. Several food nutrients are considered antioxidants, including vitamins A, C, and E, as well as the vitamin
A precursor, beta carotene. Vitamins B1, B2, and B6 are also
thought to have antioxidant properties, in addition to niacin,
niacinamide, PABA, and pantothenic acid. Certain amino acids
and minerals, such as zinc and selenium, also fall into this category. A free radical scavenger enzyme called superoxide desmutase
(SOD) also serves as an effective antioxidant. Research done by
Stephen A. Levine has shown the value of germanium (a trace
element) as an antioxidant and immune system modulator.

Dr. Abraham Hoffer, an orthomolecular psychiatrist, believes that "all people exposed to radiation should take ample
quantities of vitamin C—at least three grams per day—and quantities of vitamin E—at least 800 international units per day, as well
as selenium—200 mcg. per day." There is evidence that people
with low levels of selenium are more prone to prostate cancer
and cancers of the intestinal tract. However, selenium in large
doses can be toxic. Hair analysis is considered an objective way
of determining tissue concentrations of selenium levels.[25]

Natural, homestyle remedies may also help counter the effects of radiation. Ingrid Naiman, Ph.D., in her book, *Welcome
to Planet Earth,* suggests taking baths to which one-half cup each
of sea salt and baking soda have been added. As unlikely as it
sounds, experiments in the 1960s by researcher Frances Nixon
and a physician colleague revealed evidence that salt and baking
soda may indeed help to counter the effects of radiation.[26] Naiman also recommends miso soup as an antidote. A number of
crew members report both remedies as being helpful, especially
in combating flight fatigue.

Naiman suggests that "it is usually advisable to replace the
vital trace minerals that are leached by radiation." Liquid

supplements are more easy assimilated by the body and the assimilation process is aided by the intake of digestive enzymes or fresh pineapple juice. Try washing down mineral supplements with pineapple kefir (a yogurt-like drink) to promote swift assimilation.

In her book *Diet for a Small (Irradiated) Planet,* Robyn Seydel emphasizes the value of eating foods that act as binding agents, which rid the body of radioactive elements that we all absorb each day as a side effect of living in twenty-first century culture.[27] Since crew members and frequent flyers also receive excess ionizing radiation during flights, they should try to limit their exposure to all types of radiation including the absorbed radiation not received during flight. Seydel suggests eating a lot of fiber foods to counteract absorbed radiation, including:

- Lignins (beans, vegetables, whole grain bran).
- Gums (soluble fibers found in fruits and vegetables).
- Pectins (apples, grapes, cabbage, cauliflower).
- Cellulose (beans and whole grains).

Seydel's information is based on data presented in Sara Shannon's book *Diet for the Atomic Age.* Both note the following supplementary dietary mineral blockers:[28]

- Calcium blocks the absorption of strontium 90.
- Naturally occurring iodine blocks iodine 131.
- Iron blocks plutonium 238 and 239.
- Potassium blocks cesium 137.
- Sulfur blocks sulfur 35.
- Vitamin B-12 blocks cobalt 60.
- Zinc blocks zinc 65.

Protective qualities from absorbed radiation are also found in foods of the cabbage family cruciferae. Brussel sprouts, bok choy, chard, kale, and cauliflower, along with cabbage itself, contain the amino acids cystine and methionine. The sulfur in these amino acids has an affinity for radioactive substances that are absorbed by the body, causing the substances to combine and allowing the body to more easily dispose of the toxins. These sulfur amino acids also help to maintain healthy liver function, which expels poisons from our bodies.

The   highest   concentration   of   radioactive   particle contamination appears in milk and other dairy products, along with meat. Therefore, these foods should be consumed in moderation. Fat cells actually attract and hold radioactive particles.

According to author Robyn Seydel, sugar in the diet can increase the severity of radiation sickness. Japanese physician, Dr. Akizuki, has maintained that miso soup and brown rice helped radiation victims build immunity to the devastating effects of the Nagasaki bombing.[29]

Again, since frequent fliers are exposed to excess ionizing radiation, it is important for them to try to mitigate the effects of this and other radiation exposure including absorbed particle radiation. While many scientific and anecdotal solutions have been proposed to protect the body from all types of radiation, I recommend a high fiber diet with antioxidant supplements of nutrient vitamins for both frequent fliers and airline crew members.

Incidentally, food preparation in the air involves exposure to another form of radiation. Flight attendants use microwave ovens to heat food, despite several studies demonstrating that chronic exposure to low levels of microwaves may have a negative impact on the human heart, thyroid, brain and nervous system. Physician Robert Becker, author of *Cross Currents*, points out that "we still do not have any idea of the safe level of continuous exposure...[or] intermittent exposure from a microwave oven."[30]

Maintaining optimum health is imperative for any individual whose exposed daily to a harmful environment, especially if other lives are at stake. If one cannot avoid the radiation consequences of flying, extra health care to augment one's resistance to physical damage should be a prime objective. For more information on nutrition and flying, see Chapter 13. For more information on radiation and flying, see Understanding In-flight *Radiation: A Reference Manual,* by Robert J. Barish (available at $19.95 from IFRPS Inc., 211 E. 70th St., Suite 12G, New York, NY 10021) or Dr. Edward Bramlitt's taped 1987 address to the Aerospace Medical Association Convention ($14 from Audio Transcripts, 61 Madison St., Alexandria VA 22314).

Chapter 5

EMERGENCIES ON BOARD

In a letter to the Federal Aviation Administration, a physician described an inflight incident in which a passenger with known diabetes and hypertension became comatose-cyanotic: "The airplane had no stethoscope, no blood pressure cuff, and no emergency medications. Without these tools, I was helpless to diagnose or treat, despite such experience as an emergency physician."

Another doctor told the FAA of encountering a relatively simple medical situation that was "untreatable at 35,000 feet because of primitive medical conditions aboard U.S. commercial aircraft. A diabetic had taken his morning insulin and did not eat lunch that day. The resulting low blood sugar produced a grand mal seizure. Three physicians, all qualified to treat the emergency, were unable to provide definitive treatment because of the complete absence of any support equipment."[1]

As an air traveler, you are susceptible—especially if you are ill—to potentially life-threatening medical emergencies while flying. Yet you may not be able to receive the kind of help you need aboard a typical airliner.

Cabin First Aid Kits: How Good Are They? ✈

First aid kits aboard passenger planes began as "little more than a few bandages and splints," recalled Senator Barry Goldwater (R-AZ) at the Senate's Cabin Air Quality hearings. They were "derived from a 1924 Johnson & Johnson inflight kit now on display in the Smithsonian Air and Space Museum and based on Johnson's Airplane First-Aid Cabinet, dated 1915, twelve years after the Wright Brothers took off at Kitty Hawk." Goldwater, himself a private pilot, expressed concern not only about the airline's continued use of such elementary kits but the fact that "the crew often [does] not even know where the kit [is]."

Fortunately, in the early days of commercial aviation, flight attendants were also registered nurses. Today, attendants receive only basic first aid training. As Dr. Eve Bargmann, formerly of the Citizen Health Research Group, has observed: "untreated inflight emergencies are . . . among the leading causes of aviation related deaths in the United States."[2]

Foreign carriers recognized the need for complete cabin medical kits years ago. Some actually have three kits on board: one for obstetrical problems, another for general medical emergencies, and a third for medication. Dramatic evidence of the need to upgrade first aid kits on U.S. carriers was brought forth by a Dr. Keshishian at Senate aviation subcommittee hearings. Keshishian, a physician, cited a case where epileptic-type seizures were experienced by a passenger whose medication containers were empty. The plane was forced to make an emergency landing. Had the emergency first aid kits on board been adequately supplied, this probably would not have been necessary.

Such examples are far from unusual. Statistics in the early 1980s indicated that some 100 planes a day had to make unscheduled landings due to onboard medical emergencies, and 100 of these emergencies each year resulted in deaths. From August 1986 to July 1987, over 1,000 inflight medical emergencies occurred on commercial airlines. Since January 1988 there has been no reporting requirement for inflight medical emergencies, consequently no recent data is available.

Health activist and physician Eve Bargmann believes that

most onboard illnesses, both fatal and recoverable, are eminently treatable. She suggests that first aid kits be stocked with the following potentially lifesaving items (useful in treating shock, asthma, cardiovascular problems, seizures, and diabetic shocks): digitalis, insulin, atropine sulfate, lidocaine, nitroglycerin, aminophylinediazepam, Phenobarbital, dilantin for seizure, dextrose for insulin reaction, epinephrine, stethoscope, blood pressure cuff (sphygmomanometer), various syringes, needles, and medical instruments necessary to stop life-threatening bleeding and to save victims from choking.[3]

Expanded medical kits were not placed on all U.S. carriers until an FAA directive went into effect in August, 1986. All cabin first aid kits now must contain the following: 1 blood pressure cuff (sphygmomanometer), 1 stethoscope, 3 airways (various sizes), 4 syringes (sizes to administer required drugs), 6 needles (sizes to administer required drugs), 1 fifty-percent dextrose injection, 50 cc, 2 epinephrine; 1:1000 single dose ampoule each, 2 Diphenhydramine HCl Injection, 10 nitroglycerin tablets, basic instructions for use of medicinal drugs.[4]

While the presence of such items offers some comfort, only doctors, nurses, or paramedics who happen to be aboard the aircraft are authorized to use the items in these kits and then only upon approval of the pilot.

Up in Smoke ✈

Perhaps the most dreaded emergency you or members of your flight crew may encounter is a fire. Your crew is trained to help passengers evacuate an airplane in less than two minutes. They know that the likelihood of an explosion and/or effects from smoke may be imminent. But what if your crew is disabled by the crash or fire? Have you watched the emergency procedure demonstration or read the emergency card in your seat pocket?

A statement issued by Senator Inouye's office affirms the essential function of air packs in an emergency fire situation. "In the case of the Air Canada disaster [during the summer of 1983], it has been alleged that the cockpit crew donned their additional life-safety equipment, and believe it or not, turned off the only packs available to the cabin crew and passengers. I do not fault the crew that had to reduce fuel to the fire, but this kind of incident underscores the fragility of cabin air support systems and dilemmas which face airlines in emergency situations."[5]

The Air Canada DC-9 involved in that accident made a successful landing, but twenty-three of the forty-six occupants were overcome with toxic fumes and, unable to evacuate the plane, died in the subsequent fire.

Speedy Evacuation ✈

Smoke hoods are special head coverings that can be very effective in minimizing fume inhalation during a cabin fire situation. They provide each user with about fifteen minutes of untainted emergency air. A proposed amendment of Federal Air Regulations requiring that commercial airliners be equipped with smoke hoods for each passenger was withdrawn in 1969. One of the reasons offered for its withdrawal was the dubious allegation that donning the hoods would further delay evacuation.

In the mid 1970s, several new smoke hood designs were examined and once again the FAA concluded that they had limited utility despite the encouraging results of a test in which a cabin area was darkened before the protective hoods were donned. Evacuation time in that tryout was improved 50 percent over tests involving less sophisticated equipment.

C.O. Miller, past director of the Bureau of Aviation Safety of the National Transportation Safety Board, insists that "smoke hoods can also cost lives. On the balance, based on those I've seen and tests I've read about, I would not endorse them. You must be careful not to create greater problems while solving one [hazard] in particular." However, there are several documented cases which clearly demonstrate that had protective hoods been available, all passengers and crew might have been able to evacuate the aircraft before it caught fire.

Unused fuel released from damaged airplane tanks usually ignites into pools of fire which directly affect the damaged and open sections of fuselage. One survivor of the 1989 DC-10 crash at Sioux City, Iowa, was convinced that had smoke hoods been available, more people would have survived.

Smoke was responsible for 850 airline-related deaths

between 1972 and 1992, according to Sen. Daniel Inouye (D-HI), who in 1993 asked the FAA to require that pilot vision be assured during emergencies involving dense, continuous smoke.[6]

Federal laws require that planes be equipped with emergency exits and protective devices which allow time for escape in almost every conceivable situation. But toxic fume protection on board is nonexistent for passengers. Cockpit crew members are provided with protective masks, and only since 1990 have smoke hoods been available to flight attendants on all U.S. commercial aircraft.

The FAA says that the hoods are intended to help flight attendants fight small fires in the lavatory and cabin. But what happens if the fire becomes too extensive to smother? Chris Witkowski, executive director of Public Citizens' Aviation Consumer Action Project, believes it is absurd to provide the hoods for flight attendants and not passengers.[7]

Bertil Werjefelt, president of the engineering firm Vision Safe Inc., has presented viable, safety-promoting smoke hood designs to airline authorities since the 1970s. These hoods provide protection for both toxic fumes and sudden decompression. But airline officials claim the units are too expensive, even though they are projected to cost only 2.5 to 4.5 cents per person on a five-hour trip. The hood also weighs a mere pound. Another easy-to-use hood, designed in Great Britain, is presently available but was not being used aboard U.S. aircraft as of late 1992.[8]

The National Academy of Sciences, through its aviation safety committee, has recommended that "the FAA review the proposed rule on protective breathing devices for crew members and ascertain the desirability of supplying such equipment for all crew members, rather than limiting it to the persons expected to be involved in firefighting." In its report to Congress, the committee further recommended that the "FAA reexamine passenger protective devices and consider requiring that such equipment be available in case of inflight and post-crash fires."[9]

The FAA requires smoke hoods only for flight-crew members, to help them fight onboard fires, and most airlines appear disinterested in such devices. A small tent-like structure called EVAS was invented by Vision Safe Inc. to protect passengers and crew members alike. Capable of providing clear pilot vision even in dense smoke, it has received FAA certification, but officials at the agency echo the sentiment of several airline executives who contend cockpit smoke is too rare to justify the estimated $20,000 needed to equip a typical airliner cockpit with smoke hoods—despite the identification of smoke as a factor in hundreds of air passenger deaths over the past twenty years.

"The FAA is just waiting for another accident to happen before they take any action," says Werjefelt. Meanwhile, the Airline Pilots Association has asked the agency to bolster requirements on smoke safety equipment, and in 1991, the Senate Appropriations Committee ordered the FAA to investigate "regulations and aircraft certification requirements" that would protect pilots from obscured vision due to cockpit smoke.[10]

Smoke-Related Airline Accidents ✈

As the following examples (provided by Vision Safe Inc.) show, unsafe conditions still occur because current equipment and capabilities are not sufficient to satisfy the airworthiness requirements.

◆ [21FEB'70] American 4-engine jet transport crashed, 47 dead. Last transmissions: "...emergency we have... smoke on board I can't see anything... is crashing... goodbye everybody... goodbye everybody... reducing power we cannot see anything can you give me a low altitude?"

◆ [03NOV'73] American-made 4-engine jet transport crashed, crew died. Reports reveal: "The smoke venting system didn't work well enough to clear the cockpit in time. The plane landed 262 feet short of the runway."

◆ [31DEC'85] American-made aircraft crashed, 7 dead. Tower recording from pilot just prior to crash: "We have smoke in the cockpit! We have smoke in the cockpit!"

◆ [28NOV'87] American-made 4-engine jet transport crashed, 159 dead. Initial reports: "Pilot radios of smoke in cockpit, then silence."

◆ [11JUL91] American-made 4-engine jet transport crashed, 261 dead. Reports indicate: "...severe smoke conditions on board the aircraft shortly before the burning plane plowed into the ground at 250 m.p.h. and exploded."

Chapter 6

TOBACCO SMOKE AND

OTHER HAZARDOUS CARGO

"My chosen career as a flight attendant came to an abrupt end on July 10, 1986," Karen Thoreson *told the Senate's aviation subcommittee in a 1988 hearing on safety. "Three specialists, two in pulmonary medicine, one eminent allergist, recommended I hang up my wings. In their opinion, the symptoms I have are causally related to exposures experienced during the course of my work as a flight attendant. They believe it unlikely that I will ever be able to return to this career without recurrence of these symptoms."*

Smoking has been banned on virtually all domestic U.S. routes since 1990. Under federal law, smoking is prohibited "on any flight within the mainland United States or between the mainland and Hawaii, Alaska, Puerto Rico or the U.S. Virgin Islands that has a scheduled duration of six hours or less."

Yet there are still thousands of daily flights outside the United States which allow the deadly practice: a known cause of cancer, heart disease, and stroke. Carbon monoxide is just one of the 4,500 toxic chemicals found in secondhand tobacco smoke. Since airlines do not provide separate cabins or air-conditioning systems for smokers, every person on board inhales such toxins.

"After depositing a quantity of carcinogens into each smoker's lungs," explains Ahron Leichtman, president of Citizens Against Tobacco Smoke, "the smoke travels throughout the air-distribution system, gumming up metal tubing the same way it clogs up a smoker's arteries. We should really call this condition 'jumbo jet aneurysm'."[1]

Ozone, the potentially dangerous oxygen compound discussed previously, is a byproduct of tobacco smoke and urban air pollution. It may enter a plane's cabin through its ventilation system from the atmosphere, where it occurs naturally. The net result of passenger exposure to excessive levels of ozone and other airborne pollutants found in tobacco smoke and smog is that both passengers and crews are robbed of oxygen, deplaning in what doctor's call an "hypoxic" (oxygen starved) condition.

The No-Air Plane ✈

Both large and small aircraft have air vents and outflow valves that can, and often do, become clogged with nicotine and tars on flights that allow smoking. This may be true even on domestic flights, since the vents and valves may not have been cleaned since the 1990 smoking ban went into effect. They are so rarely cleaned that contaminated air is often trapped in the cabin indefinitely. A former employee of the Boeing Aircraft Company once estimated that 57,000 gallons of jet fuel a year were used by a typical 747 aircraft simply to haul the coagulated cigarette tar in its air-filtering system.[2] Banning smoking on all flights throughout the world would therefore result in a tremendous cost savings.

Blocked outflow valves add to the problem of inadequate ventilation aboard commercial airliners. When pilots take a "walk around" inspection of their aircraft before takeoff, the nicotine-clogged dump valves can be easily seen. I have talked with pilots who say they have never seen some valves cleaned and who guessed that if cleaning of outflow valves were done at all, it would probably only be every two years or so.

When Boeing 747s are grounded for a complete "skin" check (once every ten years) the outer surface of the aircraft is X-rayed for cracks in the fuselage and the interior is thoroughly cleaned. According to Leichtman, "one ton of debris and tobacco smoke is removed from the interior walls of the aircraft"[3] during a typical ten-year Boeing 747 inspection. It takes a lot of fuel to fly that extra payload. (These jumbo jets are primarily used on international flights, where smoking is still permitted.)

Oxygen Robbers ✈

Tobacco smoke and other cabin pollutants, along with air quality and pressure changes, contribute to oxygen deficiency (hypoxia). One senior flight attendant addressing this issue observed that "since the advent of fuel reduction measures [in the early 1980s] contamination levels seem much higher. Cigarette smoke is often unbearable and many flight attendants are complaining of symptoms related to hypoxia, such as loss of mobility, drowsiness, nausea, and headaches. Cigarette smoke contains carbon monoxide which, when inhaled, tends to preferentially replace oxygen in the hemoglobin of the red cells to form carboxyhemoglobin, and decreases oxygen utilization by the body. I observed these symptoms in myself and my flying partners. Loss of memory is accepted as normal by most flight attendants today."[4]

How Secondhand Smoke Affects You ✈

Former U.S. Surgeon General C. Everett Koop verified that passive or "involuntary" smoking can cause diseases such as lung cancer in healthy nonsmokers. Tests have revealed measurable levels of a nicotine metabolite called "cotinine" in the urine of passengers and crews in the nonsmoking areas of airplanes—up to three days after a flight.[5]

The seriousness of the impact of smoking on both smokers and nonsmokers is well known. Environmental Protection Agency studies show that a typical nonsmoker who lives or works with a smoker can inhale the equivalent of four to twenty cigarettes a day. A separate 1990 EPA report estimated that secondhand tobacco smoke each year causes 3,800 Americans to die of lung cancer and 32,000 deaths from heart disease. This is certainly a valid argument for extending a smoking ban during all air travel, not just domestic flights.[6]

Smoke in the aircraft is not only an uncomfortable nuisance

and health risk, but is also a safety factor as well. The job performance of your flight crew could mean your life. Senate testimony indicates that a pilot's competency can be eroded up to an
estimated 50 percent by secondhand smoke. Although the pilot is
behind a closed cockpit door, imagine how much the flight attendants working in the cabins are influenced by smoke.

Safety equipment is also adversely affected by cigarettes.
Sudden cabin decompression forces the immediate need for oxygen from the masks above your seat. The doors which release
these masks may be stuck in such an emergency because of a
year-old layer of tobacco tar.[7]

Smoking's Impact on Passengers and Crew ✈

Frank Buselli, a Boeing 767 pilot for a major U.S. airline, joined
his wife, Pamela, a flight attendant, in validating the problems of
smoking onboard an aircraft. In a letter to Senator John Danforth
(R-MO), the couple itemized the following cigarette-related aircraft hazards: "minor burns on hands, arms, and clothing sustained by cabin crews as a result of being brushed by careless
smokers; smoldering cigarettes dropped on floors or cabin furn-
ishings; lavatory smoke detectors initiated by smokers resulting in
crew distractions; frequent complaints from flight attendants and
passengers about 'smoky air', headaches and eye irritation; and
heated discussions between smokers and nonsmokers that sometimes require crew intervention. While these might be construed
to constitute mostly an annoyance, their frequency and distractive
nature create the potential for serious consequences."[8]

Health experts, members of Congress, American Heart Association officials, and thousands of crew members continue to
seek a complete smoking ban on all international flights. They
fear for the lives of those people who are regularly exposed to
smoky air in the cabin environment.

Frequent flier Teresa Gandhi spends lots of time traveling on
international routes and is very concerned about her health. Returning from a peace mission to Moscow and seated behind two
smokers, Gandhi was so ill upon deplaning that she was taken directly to a medical unit near the London airport for treatment.

Former cabin crew member Karen Thoresen, speaking as a

witness on behalf of a representative of the Association of Flight Attendants, related an even worse experience during her testimony before the Senate's aviation subcommittee: "In September, 1972, I began work as a flight attendant. I was in excellent health, did not smoke, and I had no family history of asthma or allergies. In 1981 and 1982, I began to notice an increase in frequency of colds, as well as in their duration and intensity. The two-to-three-day common cold became a thing of the past. I began to have recurring episodes of upper respiratory tract infection with associated bronchitis, which lasted three to four weeks, as well as a lingering dry cough."

Karen testified, "In 1982, I was treated for viral pneumonia and, in 1982, for pleurisy. In 1985, while working on a flight, I experienced chest pain in my right side, tightness in my chest, and a great deal of difficulty breathing. I asked to be released from duty and visited the emergency room at [Massachusetts] General Hospital. After a number of tests the physician on duty diagnosed the chest discomfort as pleuritic in nature without any constitutional symptoms to suggest an infection."

She said that she "was told at that time to return to flying and usual physical activity. I returned to flying, and my symptoms continued and worsened: shortness of breath both at rest and with activity, dry, scratchy throat, dry, red eyes, occasional nose bleeds, dryness along the nasal septum, headaches, nasal congestion, periodic wheezes, and inner ear fullness and pain. In my experience, most flight attendants suffer these kinds of symptoms when they fly, to a greater or lesser degree," she added.

"Cigarette smoke is a trigger that causes my problems, which are made worse by the dry air and the other fumes in the poorly ventilated cabin of the aircraft. Most of my symptoms have had acute onset either during or immediately after a flight has concluded. The symptoms progress to develop an intractable and annoying cough and/or viral infection which can persist four to five weeks. My airway problem quiets down when I am not on the aircraft...."[9]

It is interesting that Karen Thoresen's symptoms appeared during the early 1980s after deregulation, fuel price increases, and an employer decision to limit air-conditioning pack usage.

Dr. Kenneth Lyon Jones is a San Diego physician who served with me on a research committee designed to document evidence of flying and the reproductive problems of female flight attendants. Before the United States imposed limits on smoking among its domestic airlines, Jones concluded that "the most pervasive contaminant in the passenger cabin [was] cigarette smoke." He pointed out that while little specific research has been done on the impact of the airplane cabin environment on the unborn, "the accumulated data indicates the primary effect is that cigarette smoke is the number one cause for being small for gestational age in the United States today. . . . The dose relationship between prenatal smoking and childhood cancer doubles the risk for non-Hodgkin's lymphoma, acute lymphoblastic leukemia, and Wilm's tumor."

Your Right to Smoke-Free Air ✈

Patrick Reynolds, the health activist grandson of R. J. Reynolds (founder of the tobacco company which has become RJR Nabisco), has testified before the Senate's aviation subcommittee as a representative of Americans for Nonsmokers' Rights. Reynolds pointed out that there are 4,500 toxic chemicals in secondhand smoke including arsenic, formaldehyde, cyanide, ammonia, and carbon monoxide. "Breathing this toxic gas is hazardous to the health of thousands of flight attendants and a clear violation of their rights to a healthy workplace,"[10] Reynolds said.

During that same session, Ahron Leichtman asserted that "if someone came aboard a plane and pinched or slapped a flight attendant or spat upon her, the person would be removed from the plane and probably arrested. If someone brought a canister of the very same chemicals contained in ambient tobacco smoke on a plane, and sprayed them onto a flight attendant, they would be charged with assault and battery and arrested. The issue boils down to health and safety versus greed."[11]

In its 1986 airline safety report to the Department of Transportation, the National Academy of Sciences (NAS) recommended a ban on smoking on all domestic commercial flights for four major reasons: "To lessen irritation and discomfort to passengers and crews; to reduce potential health hazards to cabin crew associated with environmental tobacco smoke; to terminate the possibility of fires caused by cigarettes; and to bring cabin air quality into line with established standards for other closed environments." The NAS issued a second report that reached similar conclusions, and that same year the U.S. Surgeon General concluded that "involuntary smoking is a cause of disease, including lung cancer, in healthy nonsmokers. . . . Simple separation of smokers and nonsmokers within the same air space may reduce—but does not eliminate—exposure of nonsmokers to environmental tobacco smoke."

Hazardous Cabin Cleaners ✈

Exposure to the major pollutants previously described is exacerbated by the presence of exhaust fumes from surrounding aircraft during flight delays and volatile organic chemicals in the cabin. The latter include resins in plastic seats, walls and floor coverings, adhesives, lubricants, elastomers, sealing compounds, and coatings. Acetone, ethanol, benzene (a human carcinogen), toluene, and n-butanol are given off by these sources.

Agricultural agencies in some countries (as well as two U.S. territories) require fumigation on certain flights in order to curb entrance of harmful insects. The ventilation system is turned off and an insecticide, usually d-phenothrin (sold commercially as Black Knight Roach Killer), is sprayed throughout the cabin just before landing. Some, but not all cabin crews make a warning announcement to the passengers telling them to cover their mouths and noses. Even with such warnings, some spray is likely to be inhaled or come into contact with the skin where it is absorbed by the body.

In early 1994, the Clinton Administration began implementing a series of measures to discourage this practice, arguing that the spraying does more harm than good. The Environmental Protection Agency says the d-phenothrin used in airline cabins can create medical problems for those with allergies, asthma, chemical sensitivity, and other respiratory problems.[12]

Cabin cleaning disinfectants such as Leader Spray (which is so strong that it must be handled with gloves) and Easy Off Oven Cleaner (used in cabin galleys) are sources of chemicals to which many people are allergic, especially if they have chronic allergies. There is not sufficient time between galley cleaning and inflight cooking to burn off all the oven-cleaner fumes in order to prevent them from entering the food supplies.

Most of the cleaning agents are distributed to cabin-cleaning crews in large containers which do not show a list of their chemical contents. For example, 222L is a powerful acid soak used in toilet basins and bowls on planes that are sitting overnight, then dumped only an hour before take-off. This cleaner contains an ammonium compound, blue dye (copper sulfate), a foaming detergent, and fragrance. The components of 222L are so powerful that they can burn human skin. I recall an incident on a DC-10 when a man flushed the toilet while still sitting on it. His wife ran to an attendant and said that her husband was in severe pain—his buttocks had been scorched by the splashing chemicals. (It's wiser to stand up when flushing an airplane's toilet.)

On one airline, a small deodorizing pad called a Celeste is stuffed into the bathroom air vents so the area will smell better. The pads also block circulating air. This is not to say the pads are harmful; they simply should not be used to plug ventilation ducts.

It is hard to say how much exposure a frequent flier may receive to these kinds of chemicals and vapors since there are no monitoring systems for them.[13] One such passenger, in apparent frustration over poor cabin air quality, was observed holding his turtleneck sweater over his mouth and nose during most of a five-hour flight. When the flight attendant inquired, he told her that he was extremely allergic to whatever fumes that were present and that this was the best way for him to find some relief.

Hazardous Cargo ✈

Most passengers and many air-cargo shippers are unaware of hazardous and infectious material restrictions governing what is allowed in airline cargo bins. Some businesses facing a tight delivery schedule, will intentionally mislabel an air express package in order to avoid delay. This material will be stored in the passenger baggage compartment immediately below the passengers.

The FAA did not even begin to keep records of suspected hazardous material violations until March 1988, and the agency freely admits that there are probably hazardous materials on a majority of the more than 1,600 daily passenger airplane flights. According to a 1992 Department of Transportation estimate, flight attendants receive up to 0.13 milliSievert and flight-deck crew members up to 0.025 milliSievert dosage of radiation annually from their exposure to radioactive cargo.[14]

The situation appears to be improving, however, as some airlines now require shippers to initial a statement declaring that their cargo does not contain hazardous material. A plan was recently initiated whereby U.S. air carriers will insert warning information in ticket jackets and seat pockets describing materials banned on flights. Unfortunately, flight attendants still observe cartons with "DANGER" symbols being placed aboard conveyor belts leading to cargo bins, and research lab scientists concede they sometimes still hand-carry infectious material into the cabin.

Some products banned from baggage compartments are:

* Matches and lighters.
* Flammable liquid such as fuels, paints, and solvents.
* Flammable gases such as lighter refills and camping gas.
* Fireworks and other explosives such as signal flares.
* Poisons, radioactive and magnetic materials, oxidizing agents, and compressed gas.
* Household items and industrial products such as bleaches, drain cleaners, many aerosols, mercury, and solvents containing chemicals that cause toxic fumes and corrosion.
* Portable radios, TV, telephones, and other transmitting devices may be carried but not operated aboard the aircraft because their signals may interrupt navigation systems.

The FAA adopted a rule in early 1986 mandating that air carriers line baggage and cargo compartments with rigid fiberglass or comparable materials to improve fire resistance. This action must meet stringent fire testing standards.[15]

In 1993, an FAA official conceded that United Airlines had been granted a seven-year exemption.[16]

Hazardous Rain Repellent ✈

A rain repellent system called RainBoe is used on the windshields of many commercial airliners so that pilots can see clearly out of the cockpit during inclement weather. The liquid is similar to the various soapy mixtures that are stored in a reservoir under the hood of a car and sprayed onto an automobile's windshield.

Canisters of RainBoe are placed inside the airplane cockpit, with distribution lines running from these containers behind the instrument panel. When it rains, the material is squirted onto the windshield. In some cases, the canisters are just inches away from the cockpit crew's breathing zone.

RainBoe consists mostly of a fluorocarbon and Freon 113 solution called 1,2,2-Trifluoroethane. It also contains methylene chloride and dichloroethane, which are listed under California law as known cancer-causing agents. Reports of death as a result of exposure to chlorofluorocarbon 113 (CFC-113) and other chlorofluorocarbons have been documented by the National Institute of Occupational Safety and Health.

Information that surfaced during litigation involving a McDonnell Douglas MD-80—an airplane that leaked RainBoe fluid and its vapors—indicates that the product's active ingredient can be extremely harmful. Court documents confirm that "because of its high vapor pressure (285 millimeters of mercury) at room temperature, CFC-113 can produce high ambient concentrations of vapor during normal use of the liquid. Uncontrolled use, therefore, poses a significant hazard and can result in lethal workplace concentrations, particularly in confined spaces."

The Effects of RainBoe ✈

Overexposure to the Freon found in RainBoe has an anesthetic effect and causes deterioration of manual dexterity, loss of reaction time, cardiac sensitization and arrhythmia, and even death. A NIOSH alert requesting assistance in "Preventing Death from Excessive Exposure to Chlorofluorocarbon 113 (CFC-113)" states that "for more than a decade, published reports have indicated that fluorocarbons can induce respiratory depression, bronchoconstriction, and death in exposed workers and individuals who use them for psychophysiological effects."

The Air Line Pilots Association (ALPA) petitioned the FAA on the subject of toxic aircraft systems in 1989. In that document, San Diego attorney Tim J. Vanden Heuvel presented comprehensive documentation of RainBoe's toxicity. Yet the Civil Aero Medical Institute (CAMI), responding to an FAA inquiry, determined that the potential hazard of the chemical was small and therefore regarded it as safe. Meanwhile, a special CFC-113 warning bulletin issued by the Michigan Department of Public Health disputes the CAMI position and a National Aeronautics and Space Association study concluded that "the emergency exposure limit for astronauts [to CFC-113] should be no more than 200 parts per million for longer than sixty minutes because of its strong effects on manual dexterity and mental vigilance."

Why did the FAA certify RainBoe?

I think attorney Tim Vanden Heuvel's comment on the ALPA petition speaks for itself:

"When the system design and proprietary chemical repellent ('RainBoe') were originally certified by the FAA in 1964 for incorporation into the Boeing 727, the RainBoe chemical rain repellent was apparently believed to be, and was expressly represented to be, a 'non-toxic' and innocuous chemical. On January 24, 1963, for example, Boeing wrote to the FAA stating: 'The fluid, which is proprietary at this time, is essentially non-flammable and non-toxic.' Later, in a 'telex' dated July 1, 1985, Boeing customer support stated: 'RainBoe Type 3 is classified as inert and non-toxic.' Boeing's counsel also described the RainBoe fluid in its submissions to the Superior Court of California as 'essentially non-toxic.'"

Heuvel added, "The system design, which has numerous known leak points, some within inches of flight crew breathing zones, and its placement within the cockpit, were based upon the represented 'fact' that said 'RainBoe' was 'non-toxic.' Once the FAA has given certification approval on the premise that Rain-Boe was a 'non-toxic' and innocuous substance, all subsequent variations of the FAA-certified system, whether designed and installed by the Boeing Company, McDonnell Douglas Corporation, Lockheed, British Aerospace Engineering, Airbus, and others, a hazard mode effect analysis apparently was never considered or performed. This anomalous omission resulted from the 'sufficient similarity' procedure which allows FAA certification of subsequent aircraft systems based upon the FAA's certification of the original system without having to perform hazard mode effect analysis. As intended, and at best, this 'sufficient similarity' procedure avoids the unnecessary waste and expense of 'reinventing the wheel' and is a laudatory and desirable procedure. The potential danger of this procedure is that, at its worst, it allows the proliferation and perpetuation of an aviation safety hazard which was missed in the original FAA review and certification. [This] is exactly how the present hazard has reached such widespread status in the domestic and foreign air transport fleet. Boeing's chief toxicologist recognizes that: 'From a safety standpoint we know that this product is in a critical location in the airplane and that release of the material is possible either due to a malfunction of the product container or the distribution system itself.'"

However, action to correct the situation concerning RainBoe has not been undertaken by the FAA, despite ALPA requests for the addition of a distinctive odor to all appropriate fluids and substances in order to make quick detection easier. Installation of protective shielding and establishment of a policy ensuring that system inspections are mandatory and frequent has also been requested (and apparently ignored).[17]

Veteran USAir pilot Richard H. O'Harren was awarded $2.45 million for injuries resulting from being sprayed in the face by RainBoe windshield repellent emitted from a defective system. Persistent nose bleeds and headaches, along with abnormally high blood pressure and emotional distress, caused the pilot to miss more than a year of work. After winning his lawsuit against the companies, O'Harren was to receive $2 million in special punitive damages from USAir and $454,000 compensatory damages from Boeing, McDonnell Douglas, Dupont, and USAir.[18]

Chapter 7

FATIGUE, FLYING,

AND EVEN DYING

The men in the cockpit of Pacific Southwest Airlines' Flight 182 did not see the Cessna until it was too late. The sun was shining directly into their eyes and there was no chance to avoid the mid-air collision over San Diego that cost more than a hundred lives on a bright autumn afternoon in 1978.

Were the crew members tired and hungry? Was the flight control tower fully staffed? Was the radar tracking system outdated and inadequate? Why was a private aircraft allowed to make practice approaches at a major airport?

The lone pilot felt that he had not received adequate training and was skeptical about the airworthiness of his plane. After crash-landing shortly after takeoff, he quit on the spot—convinced that the only "pilot error" involved was having agreed to fly.

The year was 1853 and the aircraft was a boat-shaped glider topped by a kite. The question being asked then was the same one asked today after any airplane mishap: Was the cause of the accident due to pilot error, inclement weather, mechanical failure, faulty design, or a combination of factors?

One important difference between the early days of aviation and now is a dramatic increase in deadly crashes. Today's pilots have much less chance of walking away alive. In 1989—a typical year—fatal U.S. aviation accidents involved 156 commercial and 2,167 general aircraft. There were also several highly publicized non-fatal incidents, most attributed to human error.[1]

Some crashes are seemingly unavoidable accidents for which no amount of advance preparation would have saved lives. Many, however, involve factors over which airline companies, government agencies, and other authorities can exercise some control. As the flying public becomes more aware of the deadly risks of poor oversight and lax maintenance, the impetus for positive change appears to be growing.

Human Error ✈

The cause of 85 percent of all general aviation accidents falls into a category called "human error," according to aviation safety expert and former pilot John Nance.

In his book *Blind Trust,* Nance and other authorities cite overworked, inexperienced, and overstressed flight crews and air traffic controllers who must deal with adverse weather conditions, airport gridlock, terrorist threats, and a lack of support personnel, along with cost-conscious airline management and understaffed maintenance crews. According to Nance, a lack of vigilance on the part of government advisors and investigators is another contributing factor. Expert Senate testimony, interviews with airline employees, airline accident reports, and federal investigatory agencies support such claims consistently.[2]

Whatever the ultimate source of cockpit error, the costs of such miscalculations are mounting. When an Indian Airlines B-737 hit a truck during takeoff in April of 1993, 82 of the 112 passengers died and twelve were severely burned. The pilots were later charged with homicide.[3]

Near Misses ✈

A *Newsweek* magazine article, "The Year of the Near Miss," described an incident in which two jumbo jets came within 100 feet of colliding with each other over the mid-Atlantic Ocean. Despite the potential for disaster, the pilots involved actually considered not reporting the incident to the FAA, apparently for fear of reprimand or demotion.[4]

"The close calls aren't reported because pilots believe if [they] admit they did something wrong, their careers might be in jeopardy," says Nance.[5]

Fearful crew members may be unaware that NASA's Aviation Safety Reporting System (ASRS) maintains a hotline for flight personnel who wish to report a "near miss" anonymously. Some 200,000 safety lapses have been reported since 1986.

In a letter to me, Vincent J. Mellone, deputy program manager of the ASRS, maintained that statistics on "near misses" in the air and on runways "can be misleading. Both of these types of events show an increasing trend over time when the absolute numbers are examined. However, as the year-to-year numbers increase, their total contribution to all ASRS-reported incidents has noticeably decreased," apparently because larger numbers of other safety problems are also being reported.[6]

Some near misses involve poor communication. In 1992, a Los Angeles-bound USAir 737 came within a thousand feet of a head-on collision with a Southwest 737 en route to Albuquerque. The incident, which happened over California's Mojave Desert, was attributed to "controller error" after it was determined that an air traffic controller gave the planes conflicting instructions.

Near misses on the ground are a serious problem, as well, with results as potentially deadly as those in the air. "Some of the most horrendous potential accidents have occurred in runway incursions," confirmed Rep. William F. Clinger (R-PA), in a Congressional hearing on the issue. "Whether you are a pilot or a passenger, the threat of being incinerated in a midair plane collision or on the runway is indeed a sobering thought."[7]

Human error may also have played a part in separate accidents involving two Dutch-built Fokker F-28 passenger planes during cold and snowy takeoffs. Twenty-four people died in the March 1989 crash of an Air Ontario plane in Dryden, Ontario. Three years later, a USAir flight went down just off New York's La Guardia Airport, killing twenty-three people. Two accidents in 1993 also may have been caused by human error, killing a total of 103 people in Zambia and Macedonia. (As a result of those tragedies, the FAA ordered special training for pilots and stressed the importance of deicing aircraft within 15 minutes of takeoff when conditions are likely to create sheets of heavy ice on wings. New FAA rules imposed in 1992 provide time charts on how long an aircraft can be allowed to stand in freezing weather without a second deicing and require that, under certain conditions, aircraft be physically inspected to make sure no ice has formed. The FAA also now mandates that commercial airliners must be equipped with a ground proximity warning system, and that commuter and private aircraft follow the same deicing rules as those imposed on larger planes.)[8]

Costs, Understaffing, and Fatigue ✈

Air traffic control technology cannot offset the unpredictability of human error in potential plane crashes. It would not have averted the August 1985 Dallas airport disaster, for example, where a Delta jumbo jet went down in stormy weather during a period of intense wind shears (violent and fast-changing air currents).

"You could have given those air traffic controllers the most sophisticated instrumentation possible," explains pilot Nance, "and I still doubt whether they would have had the gumption to order Delta to break off its approach. They would have had to reorganize the whole traffic flow into the airport and someone might have complained about how much money the diversion cost his company. Besides, the controller might not have been backed by his bosses at the FAA."[9]

Subsequent investigation revealed that two FAA Full Performance Controllers were on their meal break when the crash occurred. Apparently, they were aware of the impending thunderstorm. One wonders if those left in the control tower knew of the storm's potential severity or if they received a thunderstorm warning from the previous tower crew.

The strain of responsibility, the stress of understaffing, and the fatigue from intense concentration permeate a flight control tower. Reporter Michael Specter of the *Washington Post* once asked Philip Kain, a controller working the congested Washington-New York corridor, to describe his job.

"It's like threading a needle at 600 miles per hour," the controller replied. "Making a mistake means backing up the whole system. There are times you are so busy here that you can hardly breathe." When his shift is over, Kain said, he takes his chair with him because it is drenched with sweat.[10]

The FAA confirmed that in 1993 there had been a 5 percent increase in operational errors by air traffic controllers over the previous year. The agency found, for example, that separation distance rules were breached 757 times in the twelve months ending in October, 1993, resulting in what one official admitted were some "relatively close" calls. Some experts blamed the rising number on increased air traffic, overburdened airports, and overworked controllers. The air traffic controllers' association said up to 3,000 new controllers need to be hired to adequately meet current demand, although the FAA claims there is no shortage.[11]

Accident Enablers ✈

Smooth and professional interaction among crew members is more crucial than ever because of the large number of newly hired pilots rising from civilian ranks. Airlines can no longer draw from what once seemed like a bottomless pool of expert military fliers. Some recruits are now going into a pilot's seat with as little as 300 flight hours, in addition to the standard simulator training provided by airline company training programs.[12]

The inexperience of this new generation of civilian pilots may account for at least some of the mishaps which have recently affected commercial airliners. From January to October 1989, there were ten fatal accidents in which cockpit human error was blamed and a lack of experience played a key role. One such incident was USAir Flight 5050, on which the rudder was set in the wrong position just before takeoff at New York's La Guardia Airport. It was the First Officer's only takeoff in a Boeing 737-400 and there was no check pilot (supervisor) in the cockpit.[13] (C.O. Miller, former director of the Bureau of Aviation Safety for the NTSB, also noted that the rudder control switch on this aircraft was "very poorly designed.")

Anonymous pilot reports to the ASRS also indicate that airline mergers or fleet inconsistencies have figured in 128 incidents from 1985 to November 1989. Adjusting to new rules on cockpit procedures, checklists, position of equipment in different and unfamiliar aircraft, and sudden change in position of cockpit command are all contributors to this compromised environment.[14]

Labor Crises and Your Safety ✦

A crisis over airline management is not always a bad thing, some say, and ocassionally one is precipitated to further management aims. But the stress of such a crisis could be fatal if the changes altered airline crew judgment and response in an emergency.

Pilots respond in a wide variety of ways when the airlines that employ them become involved in layoffs, bankruptcy proceedings, and mergers.[15]

Complaints of unfair labor practices during mergers prompted Rep. Norman Mineta (D-CA), then chairman of the House Aviation Subcommittee, to introduce a "Labor Protective Provisions for Airline Employees" bill.[16]

Meanwhile, the ALPA Central Safety Committee has reminded pilots to remain in compliance with Federal Air Regulations which require training in "maneuvers and procedures that have unique task, activity, and knowledge requirements when performed in either seat" of the cockpit. This is especially important in light of the fact that recent mergers and bankruptcies have required that cockpit personnel be ready to fly any position.

Eastern Airlines pilots and their families suffered so much stress after the Texas Air/Continental takeover that a "family awareness and communication program" was established by their ALPA representatives in order to cope with "labor recycling." Similar programs have been developed for employees of other airlines involved in mergers and bankruptcies.

A study from Virginia Tech University found that Eastern pilots subjected to unstable management suffered a wide range of personal, financial, and job-related problems.[17]

Emotional Stress ✦

The multiple stresses contributing to airplane accidents are not all flight related. Crew member anxiety and concern about strikes, merger disputes, and airline bankruptcy aggravate the conditions, which can cause accidents. Threats of dismissal for calling in sick or fear of reprimand when a mechanical check calls for grounding an aircraft can compromise the health of an airline employee, thus jeopardizing the safety of a flight.[18]

One ALPA council chairman acknowledged to his union members that instability placed them under enough stress that they were prone to make errors. "Combine this with efforts to coerce you into taking an aircraft that may be 'legal' but under the given conditions may not be safe," the official said, "and you may not be safe. You have the potential for loss of life!"

Pilots interviewed for a special edition of public television's *Nova* series, "Why Planes Crash," said a lack of airline management understanding is a recurring problem. Pressure to use less fuel, for instance, may reduce a flight's margin of safety while technically operating within legal parameters.[19]

Crew and Passenger Fatigue ✈

A frequent flier or crew member's constant companion is "flight fatigue;" a common mental and physical state resulting from such multiple stresses as sleep disruption due to time zone and shift changes, constant noise and low level vibration, dehydration, high altitude radiation, ozone poisoning, irregular eating patterns, and attempts to cope with these conditions through the use or abuse of alcohol and drugs.

After extensive research on sleep deprivation, pilot Bill Price and his colleague Dr. Dan Holley of the department of biological sciences at San Jose State University (which provides aviation research data to NASA), concluded that a great number of airplane crashes may have resulted from crew fatigue.

One of the most devastating of those accidents occurred in San Diego when Pacific Southwest Airlines (PSA) Flight 182 (a Boeing 727), collided with a Cessna 172 practicing approaches at Lindberg Field, the city's highly-congested commercial airport. This midair collision not only killed all aircraft occupants but seven people on the ground, demolishing suburban homes in its wake. Emergency crews were so shaken by the carnage that they required psychiatric counseling afterward.

Holley and Price note in their analysis of the San Diego crash that "visual identification of aircraft is the pilot's primary means of avoiding traffic in good weather conditions. In the case of PSA Flight 182, the ability to see the Cessna was greatly reduced because of exogenous physical obstacles, such as looking into the sun, color blending of the target aircraft into the background, and lack of clear visibility due to the angle of observation and small relative speed difference."

The cockpit tape recorder of Flight 182 revealed a conversation between a flight attendant and the captain of this flight that lends credence to this theory. "I'm draggin,'" the PSA pilot is heard complaining. "It was a short night."

It was confirmed that the crew only had about five hours of sleep time at layover points on both nights before the crash. According to Holley and Price, most people will feel sleepy for the entire day following a night of only five hours sleep.[20]

Fatigue and Judgment ✈

Captain Price estimates that, when fully rested, he and other pilots can react within six or seven seconds to a typical inflight emergency. "Unrested," he cautions, "we need as much as fourteen seconds to react. At the tremendous speeds of modern aircraft, fourteen seconds is too long both to solve a problem and react to avoid disaster."

The FAA's Advisory Circular 90-48C allows that it might take as long as twelve and one-half seconds to "see-and-avoid" a midair collision. The key is target size. When combined with blind spots, empty space myopia (nearsightedness), background clutter, low oxygen levels, and other debilitating factors, it becomes evident why "see and avoid" no longer works. The closure speeds are too high and the targets are too small.[21]

Crew coordination and mental acuity have sorely tested experienced pilots as well. One example is a Northwest Airlines crash in Detroit where 148 passengers and six crew members were killed. It was learned that the preflight checklist had not been performed and the wing flaps were not properly set.[22]

During the 1980s, hospital-based aeromedical helicopters had their worst accident rate in modern aeromedical history. Their crew members say they are overworked and suffer from extreme fatigue. They must also cope with stress, the pressure of a lifesaving mission, and a lack of crash protection.[23] Their record seems to have improved more recently, with only three accidents reported in 1991 and two accidents in 1992.[24]

Captain and author John Nance recalls that when he used to fly a DC-8 on the eleven-hour flight from Los Angeles to Santiago, Chile, he would "have to struggle to get sharp enough to handle the landing. You feel as if you are being flown by the airplane, not the other way around. . . ."

Fatigue may sometimes override weather conditions as the prime element in an airliner accident. Windshear is believed to have caused the August 1985 Delta jumbo jet crash in Dallas, but other factors may also contribute to such a disaster. "No pilot can justify flying into a thunderstorm," Nance maintains. "What you do is avoid the hell out of it. Delta is a superlative airline, but these pilots were overconfident of their aircraft's ability to fly through anything and they forgot some of the basics."

Did they forget these "basics" because of compromised health or fatigue? Unfortunately, we will never know.[25]

Thankfully, the intense winds implicated in the Delta disaster have become the object of increased scrutiny by scientists, who sometimes refer to them as "microbursts."

These elusive and sudden surges of energy "are the largest source of air carrier death in the United States," meteorologist John McCarthy told *Science* magazine in 1987. He estimated the winds were responsible for a combined 398 deaths in the preceding twelve years. Doppler radar systems using laser and microwave technology are now being used in 106 U.S. airports to detect windshear conditions, and the FAA is developing a pilot-training program using simulated microburst conditions. Because the wind patterns are so erratic and powerful, however, no detection system is considered foolproof.

Complete and Alert Communication ✈

Lack of proper communication has been cited as a possible factor in the 1990 crash of Avianca's Flight 52 as it approached New York's Kennedy Airport. There were long delays due to fog that cold January night. The captain had instructed his copilot to radio the flight control tower for emergency consideration to land, but the copilot asked for "priority" rather than "emergency" clearance. There are two towers involved in an approach to Kennedy and it is not certain that even the less urgent "priority" request was ever transferred to the second control tower. It now appears that many people were inattentive as a crisis situation developed. The plane simply ran out of fuel and crashed. The only saving grace was the fact that a fire did not occur because the fuel tanks were completely empty.

Hours of Boredom and Moments of Terror ✈

In a chilling 1985 incident, the crew of a China Airlines 747 battled to regain control of their plane after it rolled three times in the air and fell 30,000 feet, tearing off pieces of the tail section and bending its wings. Crew members, who had become mesmerized by their computer screens after staring at them for ten hours, forgot that they, too, could actually control the aircraft. It was not until the auto-pilot was switched off and the captain took the wheel that the free-falling plane could be righted.

Complacency and the physical impossibility of monitoring cabin control panels for long periods of time are a common problem aboard commercial jets. Crew members are now asking for electronic monitors to keep an eye on the computer-based automation equipment that does much of the "drudge work" of flying. At the same time, airline officials are asking cockpit crew members to fly manually at least some of the time in order to maintain their flying skill, despite a possible increase in fuel costs during hands-on flying.

Pilots, speaking anonymously, have expressed their concern about incidents involving automated cockpits that have stemmed from boredom and sleepiness. Former NTSB chief Miller addressed this issue when he described how one cockpit crew, given a runway change, was so busy reprogramming their onboard computers that the aircraft nearly flew into the ground. He recalled how members of another crew, while climbing to cruising altitude, noticed a severe drop in airspeed and only averted a stall when manual operation was engaged. In yet another instance, one airplane computer directed a descent while another computer engaged a level-off position and a third reduced engine power for the descent, thus reducing air speed. Once again, the pilot was able to avoid a stall by returning to manual operation.[26]

Members of the cockpit crew, who admitted to Rivera that they were asleep during crucial moments of the flight, missed its first approach and had to circle the field a second time in order to land.[27] The author recalls an incident in which all three cockpit crew members had fallen asleep as their plane approached the Saigon airport in Vietnam. In a 1991 television news special, reporter Geraldo Rivera interviewed pilots who said that they had also fallen asleep during flight.

The Aviation Safety Act of 1988 amended Federal Aviation Regulations calling on the FAA to research the relationship between human error and aircraft accidents, as well as cabin air quality and similar equipment-related safety issues. During the following five years, however, few results were reported.[28]

Alcohol and Flying Don't Mix ✈

NBC-TV's "Nightly News" reported in March 1990 that all three members of the cockpit crew on a Northwest Airlines flight from Fargo, North Dakota, to Minneapolis, Minnesota, faced state criminal charges for flying while intoxicated. The captain showed a blood alcohol level of .12 above the acceptable limit for driving a vehicle while intoxicated (for which he had a past record). The other two crew members tested at .08 and .04 respectively, which is above the limit allowed for flying. The flying certificates of all three pilots were subsequently revoked.

Drinking among private pilots can also pose a threat to commercial airliners, since intoxicated fliers may collide with larger aircraft. A 1992 NBC-TV news report estimated that 10 percent of civilian plane crashes in the 1970s and 1980s were due to alcohol or drug abuse. According to NBC, from 1983 to 1988, the deaths of at least thirty-five private pilots were linked to drinking or drugs.

The U.S. Air Force School of Aerospace Medicine previously conducted psychological and psychiatric evaluations of a large percentage of 2,700 Air Force fliers. The most common diagnoses included adjustment, psychophysiologic, and anxiety

disorders, as well as depression and alcohol abuse. Less than half
were recommended for return to flying status.[29]

The Tired Pilot is a Grouchy Pilot ✈

According to Captain Richard Stone, "pilots have been unable to
express the 'washed out' feeling they have after completing a series of flights that takes them away from home for as long as ten
days or more. Unable to explain it to others, they are often ac-
cused of being 'grouchy' and unable to enjoy the time off between trips. They experience a lassitude and lack of efficiency
that is not understood by non-pilots. When these feelings occur,
the pilots are suffering from acute fatigue. If required to continue
flying without adequate catch-up rest, they will enter a chronic fatigue phase. In short, they become candidates for accidents."[30]

In 1988, the Air Line Pilots Association called for Federal
Air Regulations defining better crew rest and flight time regulations for long-range international cockpit crew. Interim FAA
flight and duty limit rules expired in 1990 and have not been rein-
stated. Federal Air Regulations now in effect limit the hours a pilot may fly during any consecutive twenty-four hours. Airlines
can cut pilot rest periods to eight hours if the pilot is given com-
pensatory rest during the following 24 hours. Eighty-six percent
of pilots surveyed by ALPHA said they exceeded 16 hours of
duty during a 24-hour period, nine times or more per month.

In order to combat cumulative fatigue among crew members,
the FAA issued interim flight and duty time limits for two-person
cockpit crews and is supposedly revising international flight duty
time rules. In 1984 and 1985, the Association of Flight Attendants and the Joint Council of Flight Attendants unions petitioned
the FAA to set maximum duty time limits and minimum hours of
rest for cabin crew members. Their petitions were denied but the
issue came up later when Rep. Mineta introduced a bill establish-
ing maximum duty hours and minimum rest hours for flight attendants which passed the House in 1992 but failed to win
President Bush's approval. A House-Senate conference committee later deleted Mineta's provisions. The bill would also set limits on flight attendant work schedules and required that airlines
provide attendants with meals if they are on duty ten hours or

more at a stretch.[31] In some cases, flight attendants are not provided meals and are often forced to eat when the workload is excessive. This situation only aggravates stress and increases the incidence of hypoglycemia or low blood sugar among cabin crew members.

Why Do They Do It?   ✈

Crew members choose exhausting schedules which involve trips that take them away from home for five full days (and nights) a week, because they may only fly ten or twelve days a month. Many cannot afford to be away from home that long. They are helping to support their families, so they cannot quit flying; nor can they retire early because they would forfeit any retirement benefits they may have accrued.

Some of these flight attendants pick up additional flight time to earn extra money and are flying up to 140 air hours a month. Until flight and duty time limits are imposed by the government, you might very well be flying under the supervision of these fatigued crew members. Do you feel comfortable trusting your life to their response time in an emergency? Would you be able to evacuate a burning airplane without their alert help?[32]

Government Crackdown on Drugs   ✈

The air travel industry has not been immune to the escalating problem of drug abuse. T. Allan McArtor, former chief administrator for the FAA, put flight crews on notice: "If you are not drug free," he warned, "if you are not technically proficient, if you cannot demonstrate your skills, you will not fly in the national airspace." At the same time, the FAA also sent the following advisory to the executive management of every air carrier: "If you do not comply with your obligations to maintain your fleets and fulfill the obligations of your operating certificates, you will not operate in the national airspace. This goes for large air carriers as well as small ones."[33]

Electronic Gadget Hazards   ✈

Many pilots now believe that laptop computers, pagers, cellular telephones and various other high-tech electronic devices

interfere with their navigational instruments because many of
these gadgets emit spurious short-range radio signals. Studies
have validated this phenomenon and American Airlines has received as many as three complaints each month from pilots about
the problem. In 1993, Congress ordered a formal report from the
FAA about the use of electronic devices on airplanes but so far,
no action had been taken.[34]

Animal Hazards ✈

Daredevil pilot Galbraith Rogers drowned in the Pacific Ocean
after a sea gull struck his Vin Fiz airplane off the California coast
in 1912. This was the first recorded death due to a midair bird
collision. There have been two highly publicized incidents involving bird-plane collisions. One occurred in 1960 when a commercial airliner struck a flock of starlings near Boston's Logan
Airport and sixty-two people died, and in 1981 the commander of
the U.S. Air Force Thunderbird Demonstration Team collided
with a sea gull and was killed. At New York's busy Kennedy
Airport, a colony of 20,000 laughing gulls at the end of a runway
is responsible for as many as 170 bird-plane collisions annually.
In the U.S. as a whole, more than 2,000 collisions between birds
and aircraft occur each year, most in cities with low-lying airports such as San Francisco and New Orleans.

Between 1912 and 1990, at least 147 people were killed in
bird-plane collisions. Commercial airlines estimate bird-related
repairs cost them $25 million annually.[35]

Pilots also encounter other creatures in their airspace. Spiders
dangling from their webs have been tracked as high as 40,000
feet, where they occasionally meet their end in violent contact
with a cockpit windshield. In one bizarre incident, an Alaska Airlines 737 had just lifted off the Juneau runway when it collided
with a fish dropped in its path by a startled bald eagle.

On rural runways, large mammals can be a problem. Way-
ward deer are an ongoing hazard at airports in Houston and
Washington, and pilots must keep an eye out for foxes in Minneapolis and moose in Anchorage.

Chapter 8

JET LAG, SLEEP DEPRIVATION,

AND CIRCADIAN

DESYNCHRONIZATION

Life, fiscal, menstrual, and seasonal cycles. Yearly, monthly, weekly, and daily changes: we are surrounded by a sea of rhythm, vibration, and season. These include the movements of earth around the sun, the moon around the earth, and the solar system through the Milky Way galaxy. Each influences the earth's subtle magnetic fields in powerful, unseen cosmic cycles.

"Biological clocks" govern many of the functions and activities of living organisms. Cells, glands, organs, and biological systems respond to these internal—and external—forces as a part of a much larger interconnected whole.

Despite the obvious impact of natural rhythms on our bodies, the scientific community has only recently come to examine the phenomenon with any degree of seriousness. But pilots have been aware of it for decades.

Wiley Post, the famous pioneer aviator, recognized and wrote about the negative impact of time zone changes on the work efficiency of pilots during the 1920s and 1930s. Dr. Ron McFarland's renowned human factors textbook of the late 1940s and 1950s also recognized this problem. As more and more travelers and flight crews began to fly long distances with the advent of commercial jets in the 1960s, the adjustment of physiological and psychological cycles to changes in lightness, darkness, and time zones became a matter of serious concern.

Conscientious companies whose employees are forced by circumstances to travel a great deal (including some airlines) now give extra rest periods to these men and women to help them maintain mental stability in decision making. For airplane crew members, military advisors, diplomats, journalists, entertainers, athletes, business people, bureaucrats, and sales executives who fly often, getting enough rest is still a major concern.

Thankfully, extensive research is now being conducted in chronobiology: the study of the body's daily rhythm. Scientists in this field are measuring biological and chemical changes in reaction and relation to time. An allied area of investigation is chronophysiology: the study of the interrelationships among sleep, sunlight, body rhythms, the diurnal clock, and shift changes in relation to health and safety.

What is Jet Lag? ✈

When a long-distance air traveler complains of feeling "off" or mentally dull after a grueling trip, the statement is not merely a figure of speech. Laboratory tests have shown, for example, that it takes many days for the human body's steady but unconscious urinary, steroid, and electrolyte rhythms to adapt to local time after many successive and rapid time zone changes.

The term "circadian" refers to those cycles which occur in about a one day period, give or take an hour or two. Jet lag, formally known as circadian desynchronization, is caused by the rapid crossing of time zones in an east-west or west-east direction. (Although flying north-south may be tiring, it does not seem to cause jet lag.)

Our circadian cycles, popularly called "body clocks," are attuned to a home time zone with its familiar periods of daylight and darkness, sleeping and waking, eating and exercising, working and socializing. These daily cycles represent a synergistic combination of internal, external, and social rhythms which give us an important sense of time, place, and well-being. Most circadian cycles operate below the level of consciousness. When disrupted, however, they go out of phase with each other and their environment, producing a wide range of subsequent physical, mental, and emotional symptoms. For instance, heart rate and temperature rhythms become temporarily dissociated after a long trip. One might expect temporary changes in body temperature, respiration rate, reaction response, decision time, and subjective feelings of fatigue. However, not all physiological functions shift at the same speed.

In one survey of international travelers, 94 percent reported suffering jet lag, which has evolved into a generic term for the collection of symptoms described above. Half of these long-distance fliers believed the symptoms they experienced were severe. Their complaints included irritability, depression, poor concentration, indigestion, hunger at odd hours, daytime sleepiness, chronic fatigue, and the inability to sleep at night.

Frequent fliers who eat and sleep according to their local time zone seem to adapt more easily to frequent time zone changes. Others say they feel better if they eat when they are hungry or sleep when they are tired, no matter what the hour is back home. The latter approach may be possible for passengers but not crew members who must remain alert at all times.[1]

As a general rule, it takes the equivalent of one day at the new location to adjust to each time zone cross. This means, for instance, that someone flying from Los Angeles to Japan would take a full week to get used to the local time. Travelers heading from east to west generally adapt faster than those going the opposite direction as the body tends to adjust more readily to longer rather than shorter days.[2]

One of the most important of human biological cycles is the sleep/wake cycle, which can be disturbed by irregular flight scheduling and many continuous hours of flying. Circadian desynchronization and sleep/wake disruption adds to the many other stressors of flying, often creating a deep fatigue. This fatigue is relieved only after taking an extended leave from either east-west flying or any other disrupters of circadian rhythms.

Different strategies work for different people since each of our body clocks is unique. In an interview, actor John Travolta recalled sharing with England's Princess Diana his own prescription for combating jet lag: "Exercise as soon as you get off the plane and sleep as long as the flight was."[3] At layover points, the Russian airline Aeroflot has separate facilities with clocks, blackout curtains, meals, and sleep-wake cycles that are carefully calibrated in accordance with each of their country's major time zones to allow for better rest.

What works for a Hollywood celebrity or a Russian bureaucrat may or may not be appropriate for you. The best advice is to experiment with several anti-jet lag strategies.

How Well Do You Adapt? ✈

People vary in their ability to cope with frequent changes in time, place, and routine. Factors of personality, flexibility, age, and health must be taken into account, along with levels of anxiety.

Dr. J. Christian Gillin, professor of psychiatry at the University of California-San Diego, believes that 'night owls' adapt more easily. Research indicates that jet lag also affects extroverts less, while susceptible individuals may suffer manic or depressive episodes as a result of jet lag-induced sleep deprivation.[4]

People seem to recover more rapidly at home rather than in new or unfamiliar surroundings, so jet lag is often more pronounced on the outbound leg of a trip.

Prevention or reduction of jet lag and its effects has been given very limited consideration in the scheduling of pilots for commercial U.S. airlines. For flight attendants, however, the situation is even worse. Airline management tends to treat their jet lag concerns as invalid.

Jet Lag Coping Strategies ✈

There are no easy remedies for the interrelated problems caused by jet lag, circadian desynchronization, time zone changes, and exhaustion. Sheer willpower and determination will not overcome them. The best suggestions involve working to improve adaptability, building resistance to stress, and paying attention to food, drink, drugs, sleep, and rest. The key to overcoming jet lag, according to the most recent scientific studies, may lie in better understanding of how our brains respond to light and dark: the disruption of normal light/dark rhythms caused by long-distance flying appears to affect production of neurotransmitters that, in turn, affect our moods and energy levels.[5]

Some airlines take this problem seriously. Air New Zealand, for example, provides first-class and business-class passengers with an "after-flight regulator kit," containing blends of plant-based oils designed to help one either fall asleep or stay awake.[6]

Most importantly, one needs to know their own body and respond to its signals. If you have time to plan your trip, look at a map to find out how many time zones you are going to travel through. Look at your flight schedule to find out what the local time will be when you arrive. Most international flights are scheduled to land during daylight hours, based on the assumption that the activity you encounter will make you feel more awake. This is not necessarily true since your body clock may be preparing you for sleep. To prepare, try the following:

- If you will be flying from east to west, prepare by going to bed and getting up one hour later each day for every hour gained in time difference. For example, if your destination is six hours earlier (as in traveling from New York to Honolulu) you should start the new sleep pattern *six* days before leaving. In preparation, go to bed at your regular time but get up one hour later. Stay up for a few minutes to simulate your being in the new time zone, then go back to bed and arise one hour later the same morning. Do this for six consecutive days, increasing the time that you get up by one hour each day.

- If you are going to be flying from west to east, go to bed and get up one hour earlier each day. For example, a trip from Denver to London crosses seven time zones, so you should begin preparing *seven* days before departure.

   Again, start to condition yourself by pretending to go to bed earlier for the seven days prior to your trip. Lie down for fifteen minutes or so to adjust to the prospect of going to sleep, then arise. In the morning, get up at the new time and walk around for a few minutes. You can then go back to bed until your usual arising time.

- During a long flight, eat lightly (snack; do not starve yourself). Avoid alcohol, tobacco, and caffeine, and sip water or juice on a continuing basis. (Remember, if you are allergic to chemical preservatives and antibacterial sprays, bring your own food and water.) Do simple stretching and flexing exercises in your seat.

Onboard Exercise ✈

The cramped quarters of an airplane cabin are a far cry from a gymnasium or health club, but passengers may be surprised to learn how much physical exercise they can get onboard a long flight. The potential benefits of such activity are immeasurable. Keep in mind that:

- Any movement increases blood flow, thus stimulating a sense of psychological well-being and physical comfort
- Muscles and joints stiffen after periods of inactivity, resulting in fatigue, tightness, and even pain
- Simple stretching induces muscle relaxation and flexibility

Stretching of the neck, face, arm, hand, leg, and feet muscles is especially recommended during flight. For best results, combine back and forth or circular movements with deep breathing. Strengthening exercises such as lifting your body out of your seat by holding on to the armrest and pushing upward, stimulate blood flow and relieve stiffness. Try tightening and releasing sets of muscles in the buttocks, thighs, and shoulders. Press palms together to strengthen arm and chest muscles, and push against your hand with your forehead to flex the neck. Try to get up and walk around the aircraft from time to time.

Anti-Jet Lag Diets ✈

In their book, *Overcoming Jet Lag*, Dr. Charles Ehret and Lynn Waller Scanlon suggest that people attempt to manipulate their sleep/wake response with diet and caffeine (which I do *not* recommend), as well as exercise. These researchers have found that protein foods stimulate adrenaline pathways and carbohydrates condition body clocks and encourage the onset of sleep. Their anti-jet lag program involves eating proteins or carbohydrates, fasting or feasting, and drinking coffee, tea, or hot chocolate at scheduled intervals. Ehret and Scanlon base their conclusions on studies of chemicals released in the brain and the response to caffeine in laboratory animals. The application of these study results to people has been criticized by other researchers.[7] Former airline executive Stephen F. Forsyth has developed an anti-jet lag regimen that calls for avoiding all coffee, tea, alcohol, food, and non-prescription drugs on the day of your flight. The former head of TWA's Getaway Tour program recommends consuming only water and fruit or vegetable juices on the day of travel and refusing all meal service aboard the plane. Forsyth, who has followed this approach on more than 100 transatlantic flights, believes that by suspending many functions through abstinence it is easier to "reset" the body clock upon arrival.

Finally, the Argonne National Laboratory has developed an anti-jet lag diet that one might find beneficial, but it also allows caffeinated beverages. A copy of the diet can be obtained through the Office of Public Affairs, Argonne National Laboratory, 9700 South Cass Ave., Argonne, IL, 60439; telephone (708) 972-5575. (See Chapter 13 for ways to cope with jet lag.)

Light Therapy and the Anti-Jet Lag Pill ✈

Some researchers, notably Dr. Charles A. Czeisler, have found that shift workers and insomniacs may be able to adjust their body clocks and resynchronize with properly timed exposure to periods of bright sunlight. Biological rhythms are strongly influenced by how much light the body perceives. Cortisol levels and urine output indicate that the status of a circadian cycle can be measured and the body's exposure to light timed accordingly.

These findings support light research specialist Dr. John Ott's theory that some exposure to natural sunlight each day is a valid means of coping with the stress of jet lag. For example, if you are exposed to light in the early morning hours, your biological clock advances its circadian rhythms. This is advantageous if you are flying eastward. Ott believes that ultraviolet rays are essential to one's overall health and that people should spend at least thirty minutes outdoors each day regardless of the weather. He recommends against wearing sunglasses during this exposure unless absolutely necessary. If it is impossible to go outdoors during periods of sunlight, Ott suggests, sitting next to a window through which sunlight shines directly.[8]

Natural sunlight suppresses the secretion of a hormone called melatonin which is produced by the brain's pineal gland (also called the "third eye" because it is affected by any light entering the eyeball). Melatonin levels increase when a certain wavelength of light is either not present or in short supply, as is the case during winter. High melatonin levels cause drowsiness and confusion, among other physiological changes. Fluorescent lights (such as those found in airplanes and airports) do not emit the proper frequency to suppress melatonin. Therefore, on long flights the onset of fatigue may be due in part to prolonged exposure to the standard fluorescent lights found in airplanes. The use of full-spectrum fluorescent lights in airplanes and airports might help alleviate this problem, but widespread replacement of existing limited-spectrum flourescents is unlikely to occur any time soon.

An anti-jet lag pill based on melatonin and light research is now being tested, and early results are favorable. A study by British endocrinologist Josephine Arendt found that melatonin-based pills reduced the symptoms of jet lag among sixty-one people tested by more than one half. More recently, psychiatrist Alfred J. Lewy began testing the ability of minute doses of meltonin to get disjointed circadian rhythms back on track.

Acupressure and Jet Lag   ✈

A growing number of flyers (including myself) have partially offset jet lag side-effects through an approach involving acupressure that was developed by Arizona chiropractor John A. Amaro in cooperation with long-distance flight attendants. Acupuncture principles are put to use by applying stimulation with one's own fingers (not needles) at key "meridian hoary points" at predetermined intervals that correspond to time zones in one's departure and arrival cities. Gradually, the stimulation patterns are shifted to reflect the body's changing rhythms in its new location. The technique seems to help, but is no substitute for exercise, proper diet and the use of nutritional supplements.[9]

What You Should Know About Sleep   ✈

Sleep deprivation and circadian desynchronization can occur because of stress, illness, frequent schedule changes, long work hours, night jobs, and changes in types of employment. It is well known that daytime shifts are preferable to "swing" or overnight shifts in terms of the ease of obtaining sound sleep. In fact, extra pay is usually a needed inducement to get people to perform night work. Few individuals adapt to night work and actually enjoy it. It took me over two years—after retiring from almost twenty-four years of flying—before I regained an uninterrupted sleep pattern. Incidentally, flight crews do not receive any extra compensation for working at night.

Attempts to compensate for sleep disruption by chemical means have created dependencies on caffeine, drugs, and alcohol. Psychiatrists are often called upon to treat the adverse effects of shift work on marriage and family relationships.[10]

REM Sleep   ✈

Experimental studies of sleep patterns and sleep deprivation began in the 1930s. Measurements were made of the brain waves, muscle contractions, and eye movements of sleeping subjects. In 1953, sleep was found to occur in cycles which were divided into two stages: REM (Rapid Eye Movement) and non-REM. Most dreaming occurs during REM sleep.[11] Each stage is e necessary for good health and optimum performance during waking hours.

Some time is needed for "winding down" before the onset of any stage of sleep, including REM. Your mind, emotions, and body must have the opportunity to fully relax. For air travelers, the stimulation (and occasional fear) of landing, deplaning, and general anticipation all leave a residue of nervous tension that takes a while to dissipate. This is one reason why flight attendants or "jet setters" sometimes like to go sightseeing or shopping after a long trip and burn off this surplus nervous energy.

After finally winding down, the pattern of normal sleep begins. Sleep gradually deepens, then lightens, followed by a period of rapid eye movement. This is when it is hardest to awaken the body, although the mind is very active. The combined non-REM/REM stages each take about ninety minutes and cycle through four or five times every night. However, the proportion of deepest, non-REM sleep is greater during the first half of the night, and toward morning the proportion of REM is greater. Therefore, when sleep is shortened by an early wake-up call or a steady routine of only five sleep hours a night, the REM stage is generally reduced. This has important physical and psychological effects that seem to account for the more serious symptoms of sleep deprivation. Experimental psychologist Robert Hicks has concluded that "loss of REM sleep accentuates aggression and reduces critical judgment ability."[12]

The Importance of Good Sleep ✈

Scientists are still debating the actual function of sleep and admit that much about this remarkable phenomena remains unknown. Some esoteric psychologists are even studying reports of nocturnal out-of-body travel.[13] We do know that sleep allows for physical rest and rebuilding, while also providing psychological relief from the tensions and pressures of the day, thus refreshing the brain. Directing and following the patterns of your dreams in a positive manner like the Senoi tribes has been shown to enhance the quality of both sleep and psychological health.[14]

Changing times of sleep by as little as an hour can have a negative impact on one's sense of well-being. Length and quality of sleep are related to body temperature variations. Normally, one sleeps at the end of the day when body temperature drops.[15]

In order to become fully rested, your sleep experience should be comfortable and soothing. One suggested way to facilitate sleep is to lie in a north-south position, which is in alignment with the earth's magnetic field. The use of a pure wool bed pad also seems to promote sleep.

Many cabin and cockpit crew members, as well as frequent fliers, share common complaints about the poor quality of their sleep. Here is some time-tested advice on how to get better sleep:

- Use a firm mattress.
- When you sleep on your side, bend your knees slightly. Use a small pillow under your head and another small pillow beneath the knees.
- When you sleep on your back, prop your neck and knees. If possible, carry a cervical pillow with you.

- Do not sleep on your stomach.
- If the hotel bed is too soft, ask for a bed board or make a pad out of blankets and sleep on the floor.

Fatigue and Performance   ✈

Fatigue is a vague symptom not easily measured in scientific research, except as muscle fatigue. However, a decline in performance in either laboratory or real-life tasks is measurable and quantifiable. Therefore, instead of fatigue, researchers use the term "performance decrement" as a measurable result of sleep loss or deficiency. It has been scientifically verified that sleep loss and/or circadian desynchronization can result in performance decrements in areas such as: short-term/recent memory, task sequencing, attention span, concentration, visual acuity, susceptibility to error, judgment and decision making, reaction time, readiness for mental performance.[16]

Add to this list subjective symptoms such as: fatigue, sleepiness, insomnia, mood alteration, irritability, anxiety, increased neurosis, gastrointestinal complaints, headaches, nightmares, lack of appetite, feeling of disorientation, loss of sense of time, decreased libido, female reproductive system problems.[17]

Task Complexity, Vigilance, and Alertness   ✈

For cockpit crews, takeoffs, descents, and landings are the most stressful part of any flight. They require the most vigilance and mental alertness, as well as a fast reaction time. In between, while flying long distances (especially at night), pilots are mostly monitoring equipment. This is a complex but essentially boring task. If something unusual should occur, vigilant and prompt decision-making may not be forthcoming among members of a sleep-deprived crew.[18]

Cabin attendants are more physically active than those in the cockpit and presumably less subject to boredom. Nonetheless, they have added stress factors with which to cope. An emergency or unusual situation places an increased demand on an exhausted flight attendant who may not respond correctly.

Cockpit and cabin crew members tend to take naps during layovers to make up for lost sleep. Naps may reduce performance decrement for a short time, but they are no substitute for regular sleep since they may not contain a sufficient number of REM or non-REM periods.

Astronauts orbiting in the perpetual twilight of space say they nap instead of sleep for hours at a stretch. The intervals of napping coincide with their normal sleep schedules back home and a sunlight/shadow cycle replaces the day/night intervals. Just think of what this would do to your own sense of place and time![19]

Insomnia ✈

Insomnia is a common sleep problem among frequent fliers who often do not get necessary sleep. For this reason, alcohol and sleeping pills are often used to induce sleep. Both alcohol and barbiturates depress REM sleep and are addictive. The resulting dependency has a detrimental affect on performance and can create personality disorders, not to mention liver damage.

Hypnotic drugs such as Valium and Dalmane are found to impair memory and reduce performance of skilled tasks the following day. The half-life of some hypnotics is fifty-four hours. Other non-hypnotic drugs cause problems as well. Even nicotine addictions interfere with deep, restorative sleep.[20]

The Hazards of Caffeine ✈

Caffeine is found in coffee, tea, soft drinks, chocolate, pain relievers, cold remedies, and various "legal" stimulants. It is a drug often used to increase wakefulness. This can be useful if you are sensitized to the substance, but constant use has a disrupting effect on sleep that corresponds in proportion to the amount consumed. The herbs kola (from which cola is extracted for soft drinks) and guarana contain caffeine without the acids found in coffee beans. Their addictive properties, however, are the same as coffee. Caffeine is known to cause sleep pattern disruptions.[21]

Chapter 9

FLEET FATIGUE: THE CLEAR AND PRESENT DANGER OF AGING PLANES

The roof of an airplane peels away. A flight attendant is pulled out by the sudden decompression and falls 24,000 feet to her death. Another flight attendant, Michele Honda, actually pulls herself back inside the aircraft, then helped the third attendant in protecting the ninety-four passengers while the cockpit crew guides the fractured Aloha Airlines 737 safely to the ground.

Flight attendant G.P. Lansing is later given posthumous honors, but unanswered questions remain about the tragic incident that took her life. Did inspectors alert the Federal Aviation Administration (FAA) to the serious structural weaknesses in this aged airplane? Why, as Laura Parker reported in the Washington Post, *had the FAA "cited Aloha for not having an adequate auditing system to assure that its jets were properly maintained."[1]*

Complaints about aging passenger aircraft have been commonplace as far back as the 1950s when safety concerns surfaced about the first commercial jetliner, Britain's Dehaviland Comet. Today, old and dilapidated aircraft are widely viewed as a major threat to passenger health and safety.

The *Encyclopedia of Aviation* defines metal fatigue as "failure caused by repeated stress. A ductile metal (such as steel or aluminum) is somewhat flexible, but when forces pushing against it are removed, metal returns to its original state. Beyond a certain stress, however, the deformation is permanent, and eventually a point is reached when the metal will fracture."

Aloha's Boeing 737—"old #52"—had the classic symptoms of fatigue. It was nineteen years old, had made 89,680 flights, operated in a very damp and corrosive climate, and was pressurized for as many as eight or nine landings every day.

In 1992, an investigation determined that an El Al cargo jet involved in an October crash had experienced a midair engine fire just two months earlier. Forty-three people were killed when that same Boeing 747 engine, along with a second engine, fell off over an Amsterdam suburb. A Boeing official told reporters he believed "burned" (corroded) and fatigued fuse pins, the critically important bolts that keep engines attached to the 747's wings, may have been at fault, as was the case in a 1991 Air China accident. After the Netherlands disaster, the FAA ordered replacement of all older 747 fuse pins and inspection of newer pins.

Another mechanical mishap occurred on a Kuwait Airways flight ferrying former President George Bush. But metal fatigue is not the only problem. In a CBS-TV newscast, Peter Greenberg disclosed that so many items were removed as souvenirs from the plane commandeered by hijacker D. B. Cooper that the airline changed the insignia so passengers would not recognize it.

"I believe the most serious and potentially volatile problem facing aviation today is the number of older aircraft in the commercial aircraft fleet," Rep. Dan Glickman (D-KS) told Knight-Ridder reporter James R. Carroll in a 1988 interview. Glickman later introduced a bill that required that the FAA carry out a regular dismantling of aging aircraft in order to locate cracks and corrosion in inaccessible places. In 1991 it was signed into law as the Aging Aircraft Safety Act.

Factors Contributing to Aircraft Aging ✈

Airplane aging is related to the number of hours flown as well as the number of landings and takeoffs, which involve multiple pressurization and depressurization changes. Humidity and other climatic conditions are also important contributors as is, to some extent, chronological age.

With so many parts involved in such a complex mechanism, airplanes represent many opportunities for disaster. Seams, for example, can split during flight. "Cold bonding" is a process that was used to join seams to the metallic skins of earlier 737s, 727s, and 747s. In 1972 Boeing discovered this adhesive could also come apart, so the manufacturer discontinued its use. Boeing issued a bulletin to airlines advising them of this problem, and then updated the alert just two weeks before the Aloha tragedy. In its advisory, Boeing recommended visual inspection followed by sophisticated electrical tests when cracks were found.

An investigation of the Aloha accident revealed no evidence that the electrical testing ever took place. On May 23, 1989, NBC-TV's "Nightly News" reported the National Transportation Safety Board's finding that Aloha did not supervise the maintenance program correctly nor did the FAA enforce the airline's lack of compliance.[2] Under federal law, a plane's structural, mechanical, and electrical components are to be thoroughly inspected after every four to five thousand hours of flight. If a major structural problem is noted during this so-called "D" check, other carriers with similar planes are to be alerted through service bulletins and FAA airworthiness directives.

Air Line Pilots Association officials do not believe this procedure is adequate, but the FAA feels developing a more comprehensive reporting system would be too costly and would not necessarily improve safety. Officials have said the agency needs more money to pay for more inspectors.

The FAA has been criticized for not providing enough inspectors for the periodic examination of airliners. The agency, in turn, terms its inspection program "extensive" and "designed to detect discrepancies prior to failure. Additional procedures...provide additional safeguards."[3]

Aircraft inspection practices vary with each airline, depending upon appeals made to the FAA regarding the geographic environment of planes, types of flight operation, and other factors. In going through this series of appeals, an airline can adjust maintenance procedures and intervals established in the manuals of the FAA's Maintenance Review Board. In reality, no FAA directive says airlines must follow the maintenance schedules outlined by the review board. There also seem to be holes in the policy for reporting maintenance difficulties. While some airlines are very safety conscious and meticulous about aircraft maintenance, others cut corners in this area, often pleading financial hardship.[4]

In November 1992 the FAA slapped Delta Airlines with a $2-million fine, saying it had violated a long list of maintenance and safety rules. Federal inspectors found, for example, that Delta had been operating the auxiliary power unit of a Boeing 737 for more than 3,000 hours beyond its normal maintenance check, and had operated another airliner on sixty-three flights while ignoring an FAA order to inspect the plane for cracks in the rudder control system. Prior to its 1991 bankruptcy, Eastern Airlines also paid large fines for maintenance neglect.

Aging Aircraft: A Safety Risk? ✈

A growing number of experts has expressed concern that the buying, selling, and flying of used aircraft by various carriers poses a serious safety risk to passengers. Lives may be jeopardized by the simple metal fatigue and normal wear-and-tear experienced by such airplanes.

In an extreme example of this phenomena, CBS-TV reported in 1992 that an Air New Zealand plane, which once suffered a hole blown out of its side, had been repaired and was being flown by United Airlines.

In an extensive Dallas *Morning News* article on the subject, FAA official Jim Hart told reporters David Tarrant and Ed Timms that "the airlines say they simply can't afford new jets. Folks have to cut somewhere [and] maintenance is one of the most obvious places to do that. With an older airplane, those things don't match up well."

Other FAA officials note that while used aircraft sales have increased, the maintenance costs for older planes, which historically suffer more cracks and corrosion, are actually greater than for new airliners. Insurance costs for older planes are also higher.

Premiums paid by U.S. commercial carriers rose from $272 million in 1985 to $373 million in 1986. The *National Law Journal* has set a potential liability of $1.25 million per seat on planes involved in crashes.[5]

Aloha's plane was nineteen years old when its roof peeled off in midair. The average age of U.S. commercial jets is now twelve and one-half years, and it is not unusual to find aircraft in use that are twenty years old. The average age for eleven major U.S. common carriers was compiled in 1988 by reporter James R. Carroll and published in the *Wichita Eagle-Beacon*:[6] Some four years later, many of these aircraft were still flying. Reporter Tom Webb listed seven models of the oldest commercial aircraft still in operation in a shocking 1988 *Boca Raton News* article entitled "When Is A Jet Too Old To Fly?"[7]

According to a 1992 study by Avitas Inc., the average age of the fleets of major U.S. carriers as of the first quarter of that year was: TWA (18 years), Northwest (16.2 years), Continental (14.4 years), United (11.5 years), USAir (10.2 years), American (9.2 years), Southwest (6.9 years), and America West (6.6 years).

Even with the FAA's call for regular comprehensive inspection of older commercial planes, incidents are still being reported. In late 1989, for example, part of the wing of a Continental B-747 dropped into the ocean. About a month later, a Northwest Airlines plane lost power in one of its engines when water leaking from a forward toilet froze and sent ice slicing through the jet's intake manifold.

Many factors are believed to have contributed to the 1991 Avianca disaster in which a Colombian jetliner ran out of fuel and crashed near New York's Kennedy Airport. It is worth noting, however, that the Boeing 707 involved was twenty-three years old and had been in maintenance for repairs thirty-seven times in the four months preceding the tragedy.[8]

Although a federal court found Pan American Airlines negligent in the Lockerbie, Scotland, crash of its Flight 103, the families who filed claims against Pan Am have received nothing from the court's multi-million dollar award. However, a segment of CBS-TV's "60 Minutes" news program reported that Pan Am and U.S. Aviation Underwriters' Insurance Co. have paid a detective $200,000 to investigate the disaster. The unnamed investigator claims that the CIA, allegedly involved in a drug subplot, is responsible for the tragedy. The CIA labeled the accusation reprehensible and insisted it has no validity. Meanwhile, some people in the airline industry believe that Pan Am filed for bankruptcy in order to avoid paying any claims.

Bogus and Defective Airplane Parts ✈

Interviews with former FAA inspectors and other expert witnesses on the May 19, 1990, edition of CBS-TV's "60 Minutes" program and a May 5, 1992, segment of NBC-TV's "Dateline" revealed that major aircraft manufacturers and concerned carriers are frustrated in their attempts to convince the FAA that faulty aircraft replacement parts are an enormous safety problem.

Substandard parts are obtained from stolen planes, military auctions, surplus or scrap piles, as well as many distributors, brokers, and jobbers who cut corners in order to save costs. Even parts from crashed airplanes have been used, implicated as the cause of serious accidents and incidents in other aircraft.

According to NBC, a 1985 Midwest Express DC-9 crash in Chicago—originally blamed on pilot error by federal inspectors—may have been caused by a faulty part that had been improperly installed. It was determined that a small device in the right engine, called a spacer, had cracked and shattered into many pieces. Investigators discovered that this item had been repaired improperly by a Miami parts shop rather than the airline's own facility. Harry Schaefer of the Department of Transportation said he felt that the faulty spacer should have been scrapped instead of rewelded into the DC-9.

Later, a United Airlines mechanic discovered a counterfeit spacer aboard one of the carrier's airliners that might have caused the same kind of accident as that experienced by the Midwest Express plane. In 1992, the same Miami parts shop implicated in the Chicago crash was found to be shipping faulty jet engine starters to several major airlines, possibly including United.

All overhauled parts are supposed to carry a "yellow tag" with the signature of an FAA-licensed mechanic certifying that the part is free of defects. William Gavin, head of the FBI office in Miami, told NBC in its "Dateline" report that these certification tags are sometimes counterfeited. Tom Coffee, in the airline repair business for over twenty years, said that yellow tags were routinely faked by an airline repair shop that he worked for. A subsequent FBI probe forced the offending company out of business, but the FAA subsequently certified a new facility run by the same owner even though the regulatory agency knew that he had previously run a bogus parts shop. This company is now licensed to provide parts and repair planes for all major airlines.

The Aerospace Association's Bogus Parts Committee believes that throughout their industry, parts are being used without proper examination to ensure their airworthiness. The FAA claims it is powerless to do anything about this situation and that it has no jurisdiction over such middlemen.

When Anthony Broderick, the FAA's assistant administrator for regulation and certification, was asked by "60 Minutes" as to how often he heard about the existence of a bogus part, he replied: "Two or three times a month." But he went on immediately to contend that bogus parts do not affect air safety.

"There has not to my knowledge," Broderick insisted, "been a single accident in the last ten to twenty years as a result of a bogus part in a civil aviation accident."

However, "60 Minutes" found government computers showing sixty-one accidents between 1976 and 1989 related to or caused by bogus parts. Most of these accidents involved small aircraft, executive planes, and helicopters. According to the same CBS report, one supplier "pleaded guilty to falsifying quality assurance tests on airplane nuts and bolts." This particular company claimed "to have had fasteners in almost every plane that flies."

The FAA was assigned part of the blame (along with McDonnell Douglas and General Electric) for the defective mechanical part (a titanium fan motor disk) that caused the 1989 crash of a United Airlines DC-10 in Sioux City, Iowa. *Aviation Week & Space Technology* magazine reported that the fatigue-crack in the disk was overlooked in a 1988 in-service inspection.

In the first six months of 1992, the FBI and the Department of Transportation confiscated almost 200 cases of bogus airplane parts. Although there are many highly respectable parts manufacturers, the criminal element has definitely crept into the business. How long will it be before yet another airline disaster is attributed to a used, stolen, or bogus part?[9]

New Planes Can Be Hazardous, Too ✈

Just because an airplane is new does not necessarily mean it is any safer than an older model. In 1991, for example, California-based manufacturer McDonnell Douglas conducted tests on its new MD-11, a wide-body passenger jet. The company first discovered that the plane was going to have up to 7 percent less range than predicted, but revised the seat plan to hold 410 passengers instead of the original 287. Dozens of people were injured (including a sixty-year-old woman who became paralyzed when her spine was broken) during drills conducted to see if the reconfigured MD-11 could be evacuated within the ninety second maximum time set by the FAA. Needless to say, the plane failed the safety test. McDonnell Douglas subsequently chastised the FAA for setting strict rules regarding realistic evacuation conditions and sought safety certification through computer simulation.

Star Crazing ✈

An unusual phenomenon on airplanes called "star crazing" is also cause for concern. Crazing is the result of pitting and cracking caused by encounters with sulfuric acid released into the stratosphere by volcanoes, occurring primarily in the northern hemisphere. During winter months near the poles, these incidents can take place as low as 20,000 feet.

Star crazing is the reason for almost constant replacement of acrylic passenger and cockpit side windows. (The cockpit's front windows are made out of more durable tempered glass.) Airline officials claim that "crazing" is only an expensive nuisance and not a safety problem because they believe the effect on other airplane parts is minimal.[10] However no thorough study has been carried out to back up this assertion.

Chapter 10

HEALTHIER FLYING:

HINTS FOR FREQUENT FLIERS

AND CREW MEMBERS

Pat, a flight attendant for thirty-four years, remembered being pulled over by a police officer for weaving as she drove home from an airport after an exhausting overseas work assignment. "He thought I was drunk," Pat recalled, finally able to laugh at the experience. "I fell asleep while he was writing the ticket!"

People who fly often face a bewildering array of special health risks associated with air travel. A number of steps can be taken by these individuals to reduce their chances of becoming ill, inconvenienced, or injured as a result of flying. In the long term, however, the cooperation of the aviation industry and government regulatory bodies will be required if risks such as radiation exposure and cabin air quality are to be addressed adequately.

For instance, airlines could substantially reduce the number of sick days claimed by crew members if proper amounts of rest were provided in the first place. With a subsequent reduction in stress and fatigue, employees would be happier, more efficient, and less prone to making potentially fatal errors.

But plenty of things can be done on an individual basis.

Iron ✈

At high altitudes, your blood needs more red cells to carry the smaller amounts of oxygen available. If your body is anemic (lacking in iron), you cannot build the additional cells that are needed. Hypoxia (a lack of sufficient oxygen) may increase iron absorption, and constant exposure to low oxygen environments contribute to anemia.[1] If you are anemic, it will be harder for you to function energetically unless you correct the problem.

Iron-deficiency anemia is not alleviated by taking iron supplements alone. In order to absorb iron, one needs adequate hydrochloric acid in the stomach, vitamin C in the bloodstream, and sufficient amounts of calcium, protein (especially lysine), copper, vitamin B12 and folic acid elsewhere in the body. A lack of vitamin B6 and zinc can mimic the symptoms of anemia.[2]

Hypoxia ✈

Cabin crews work in a "smog zone" of pressurization, pollutants, and both human and mechanical activity. This causes both them and passengers to suffer from hypoxia, a deficiency of oxygen.

Insufficient oxygen in the blood can alter judgment significantly. Therefore, when a flight attendant becomes hypoxic, he or she may not be able to recognize his or her own modified behavior in time to ask the cockpit crew to adjust the flight's altitude and/or turn on all air conditioning packs, both of which would pump more oxygen into the cabin. Airlines need to provide better training so that crews can recognize these hypoxic symptoms.[3]

Foot and Leg Care ✈

You may have noticed the tendency of feet and ankles to swell considerably while flying. This can be caused by cabin pressurization changes and/or edema. Paying prompt and proper attention to this condition may save much pain later on.

Properly fitted shoes are essential for flight attendants and any frequent flier. Shoes with cushioned soles and arch supports, preferably custom-made, will greatly improve one's comfort level while flying. After a day on your feet, try rubbing them with petroleum jelly, castor oil, or olive oil (with some vitamin E added). A foot bath will also soothe and refresh weary feet. A hot cider vinegar pack and oil of sage, foot soap, or foot therapy powder can be helpful, as well.

Alternating ice packs and hot water often relieves aches and pains, while foot massage and reflex therapy helps the whole body feel better. Some believe support hose helps prevent leg aches and swelling. It is always a good idea to prop your feet up whenever possible.

Some airline dress codes require female attendants to wear two-inch heels, setting up ideal conditions for back pain, internal organ displacement, and accidents due to falling or tripping. Correct posture and walking affect the entire body. If your feet hurt, you often ache all over.[4]

Eye Care ✈

When a group of Boeing 747 flight attendants was questioned about eye problems they experienced while flying, a surprising 95 percent reported discomfort, redness, and dryness. This was the case whether or not they wore contact lenses, although lens wearers seemed to suffer more, apparently due to low humidity and airborne pollutants in the cabin. Nonconstrictant wetting drops help alleviate this kind of eye irritation.[5] My own ophthalmologist suggests using moisturizing drops every hour when flying whether or not one wears contact lenses.

When there is a decrease in air pressure, as in an airplane cabin, the eye expands and presses tightly against contact lenses that have been fitted at elevations at or near sea level. Lenses fitted at higher altitudes such as Denver or Albuquerque (both around 5,000 feet) may be more comfortable. Consult your ophthalmologist for advice on how to respond to this phenomenon.

Excessive Noise and Vibration ✈

Researchers have verified that exposure to continuous and nondescript low-level sound (called "white noise") can cause severe physiological and psychological strain. Ongoing exposure to steady or continuous noise seems to be the single greatest contributor to hearing loss.[6]

Surveys taken by air-safety committees found that more than

51 percent of flight attendants questioned had suffered some degree of hearing degradation, usually involving higher frequencies. The severity of loss depended upon individual sensitivity, the type of noise, and length of exposure. These results come as no surprise to cabin crew members. A flight attendant responsible for opening a door or dropping stairs on an aircraft when the engines are running is in danger of being exposed to sound levels capable of damaging human hearing. Earplugs are one obvious and worthwhile strategy for dealing with this situation.

Some airlines no longer require or provide hearing tests every year for their employees. It is suggested that you take a hearing test if you notice an appreciable difference in your hearing. Experts feel that many hearing disabilities may become irreversible if ignored.[7]

Most people are not consciously aware of how much noise adds to the stress that already exists in their lives. Yet sounds associated with air travel, whether one is strapped aboard a jet plane or living in a house under a flight path, are indeed important stressors. Increased noise during takeoff and landing, cruising noise, ultrasound vibration, and sudden, unexpected noises all add to flight fatigue and stress.

In the long-term, these loud sounds may also cause hearing loss. It is an established aeromedical fact that because of sustained high intensity noise, many flight crew members will suffer permanent hearing damage (particularly in the high frequency range) as a result of their work.

Loss of hearing is itself a stress inducer. One flight attendant has said she now has to sit in the front of a church or auditorium in order to hear anything. According to one expert, flight personnel can expect at least a 10 percent hearing loss over the course of a decade. This statistic applies to military pilots as well.[8]

Research has shown that a phenomenon called "whole body low-frequency vibration" also stresses the body by causing biochemical changes in calcium metabolism and altering the structure of the lumbar vertebrae. It can cause fatigue, headaches, and irritability. There are several sources of such vibrations in the operation of modern airplanes, including engines, wings, and winds. All contribute to the stress of flying.[9]

Back and Muscle Strain ✈

Back problems are a common occupational hazard for pilots, flight attendants, and frequent fliers. Working in confined areas and sitting in poorly designed seats can cause back strain, as well as more serious injuries and disorders. Passengers carrying heavy luggage and seated for long periods of time may also suffer pain. Much of the time, cabin crews are literally walking uphill and downhill as the airplane ascends and descends. Pushing, pulling, and lifting heavy food-service equipment and luggage in a limited space increases strain, as do air pressurization cycles. Certain aircraft ascend and descend at steeper angles than others, further aggravating the problem. Short-range flights may only level out for a few minutes. Even then, the aircraft can still be tilted at a five-to-twelve degree angle.

Manufacturers and airlines need to design lightweight equipment with safe, easy, and healthy operation in mind. In the meantime, all crew members should be advised of proper lifting procedures, and the appropriate amount of time should be provided for the serving of food. "We're working so fast that we don't take time to lift things the proper way," said attendant Mary Evelyn. "We're straining, pulling, and injuring muscles, especially those in our backs."

To maintain a healthy back, always assess the size and weight of the object you are going to lift. Get help if it is too heavy. Hold the object close to the front of your body, with elbows bent, and bend your knees and hips so your legs bear the bulk of the weight. Do not bend or twist at the waist.

If you hurt or strain your back, have it checked immediately. Do not continue to work when you are in pain. Many chronic problems result from back and neck injuries that have gone untreated. The pain may initially go away, however, not because the injury has healed, but because the body has adapted to the problem. As a result, some people needlessly develop osteoarthritis (common among senior flight attendants) or other serious problems related to chronic back ailments that afflict all age groups. Periodic spinal checkups are recommended for anyone exposed to back stress on or off the job.[10]

Metabolic and Pulse Rates ✈

No extensive tests have been conducted in the United States on variations among airline crew members or passengers in their relative metabolic or heart (pulse) rates. However, some information on these rates, along with cabin humidity and carbon dioxide, were collected in Japan. A researcher named Toshitada and his associates found that metabolic and heart rates were higher in actual flight than in mockups that took place on the ground. This suggests that the body tries to increase its oxygen intake in the pressurized atmosphere of an airplane cabin.[11]

Fertility and Pregnancy ✈

According to San Diego physician Kenneth Lyon Jones, "research indicates that alcohol, hypothermia, smoking, and certain chemical substances have a negative effect on the fetus." Other than medical X-rays, he reports, "there is no other exercise or work which takes more blood flow away from the internal organs and from the fetus than weight lifting, and pushing and pulling the heavy carts and equipment in flight."

Jones said that a drop in the core temperature of a fetus between the fourth and fourteenth week of pregnancy "can lead to a pattern of malformation associated with prenatal onset growth deficiencies. Flight attendants working the galleys, especially the lower galleys, are especially affected. The primary effect of hypothermia is on the central nervous system [of the child]."[12]

Alcohol and Drug Abuse ✈

Abuse of alcohol and drugs by aviation employees, particularly cockpit crew members, is a serious problem that can (and does) affect the safety of airline passengers. In belated recognition of this situation, the 1992 Department of Transportation Appropriations Act urged the FAA to establish programs for testing commercial aviation employees in safety-sensitive positions "for unlawful use of alcohol and drugs." The law included provisions for mandatory testing after fatal or serious accidents and for the establishment of employee rehabilitation programs. Meanwhile, pilots have formed Birds of a Feather, their own support group for alcohol and drug abuse (contact the ALPA for details).

Pilots and Artificial Sweeteners ✈

Pilots need to be aware that their consumption of artificial sweeteners may affect their ability to fly a plane. When interviewed by reporter Deborah Whitson on a 1990 health news special over the CBN cable TV network, several commercial airline pilots reported health-related symptoms that they felt were related to their use of aspartame, an artificial sweetener commonly used in diet drinks. These side effects included disorientation, a lack of mental acuity, migraine headaches, and even grand mal seizures. Some pilots lost their jobs as a result of the problems described.

Other symptoms have been reported to researchers and physicians by patients ingesting products containing the artificial sweetener Aspartame (found in Equal and Nutrasweet). Among the problems associated with this particular ingredient are: nervous disorders, confusion, convulsions, vision problems, memory loss, numbness, cramping, lightheadedness, and nausea.

Patients say that when they stop using artificially sweetened products, their symptoms usually disappear. The Food and Drug Administration has refused to remove these products from the market or post warnings about any possible negative side effects. When queried by crew members for guidelines about the use of these products, the FAA has deferred to the FDA.[13]

Pilot Vision ✈

Flying conditions can compromise a pilot's vision. Susan Watkins and Leona Langan of Cornell University conducted research that found that pilots who flew with tight collars were more likely to suffer poor vision and retinal dysfunction because the flow of circulation to the optical area was impaired.[14]

Pilots are also advised to use extra oxygen during night flights not only for energy, but to improve their night vision.[15]

Pilot Cancer Risk ✈

Although no hard scientific research has been conducted, there appears to be a higher than normal incidence of skin cancer among members of cockpit crews. The combination of wide windows, bright sunlight, and high altitude radiation may all contribute to this phenomenon.

Male crew members experience an increase in prostate cancer and sterility, which some believe is also flight related. Periodic checkups for all cancers are advised.[16]

Psychological Effects of Crashes and Hijackings →

When the hijacking era began—with the early 1960s takeover of a Continental Airlines Boeing 707 in El Paso—airlines and their crews were not aware of the lingering aftershock cabin employees would suffer.

At first, flight attendants involved in hijacking incidents were asked to return to their assigned schedules right away, despite the deep psychological trauma such an event can inflict. Confronted with back-to-work orders, which seemed to dismiss the six fearful hours she had just spent with a sharp knife at her throat, one flight attendant immediately quit flying.

Life magazine noted after the 1989 United Airlines disaster in Sioux City that "life seems utterly different for most of the survivors. Many of them witnessed horrors that can never be erased."[17] A 1989 article in the *Wall Street Journal*, described how flight attendant Susan White had plunged into deep despair after surviving the Flight 232 tragedy, plagued by guilt feelings, terrible dreams, and premonitions of her own violent death.

Stress from Airline Reorganization →

An air carrier bankruptcy or reorganization can cause increased stress and fatigue among pilots, flight attendants, and other airline employees, possibly to the point of jeopardizing a flight's safety.

One concerned pilot, a representative of the Air Line Pilots Association, expressed the hopelessness felt by many of his colleagues during the financial downfall of their company.

"In times such as these," he said, "it is so very difficult to forget. Animosities are built that can tear away at your soul, day after day, for the rest of your life. If you let them, these animosities will break marriages and worse."[18]

HOW TO COPE

WITH STRESS IN THE SKIES

Fed up with delays, sitting in 110° heat, and choking on the exhaust of surrounding aircraft, Captain Ray Davidson picked up the intercom microphone and informed his eighty passengers that he was "sick and tired" of the situation and was taking the plane back to its gate. When he had done so, the veteran airline pilot picked up his bag, walked off the plane, and resigned.[1]

Pilots such as Davidson are not alone in their frustration with working conditions in the air travel industry. Crew members, passengers, and air traffic controllers all suffer from the many stresses associated with flying. Stress is a physiological reaction to real or perceived physical or emotional threats. It is the human body's "fight or flight" response, evolved by nature over the millennia in order to assure survival of the individual. While in one sense stress is indeed a very natural phenomenon, its impact on behavior can have far-reaching implications, especially in the modern aviation industry.

The Stress Response ✈

The stress response mobilizes such adrenal gland hormones as adrenaline and cortisol to help the body prepare for escape and to make the muscles more sensitive to commands from the brain. As a result, the heart beats faster and stronger, the peripheral arteries contract to increase blood pressure, and the liver produces sugar from stored chemicals to give the body more energy. But problems arise when this very protective and primeval response either occurs at inappropriate times or is not completed.

Air traffic controllers, for example, have a sense of responsibility for the lives in the airplanes they are directing. But as workloads increase, their confidence may be replaced by feelings of anxiety or the sensation of being overwhelmed and out of control. Working in a state of constant alertness often stimulates, unconsciously, the "fight or flight" response among flight controllers. But in the course of their workday, such individuals neither "fight" nor "run away" from the source of their nervous energy. Therefore, the physical changes in the body, which prepare them for these reactions, are never resolved. Blood pressure remains high due to the effects of stored glycogen, hearts beat faster because of adrenaline, and blood sugar is poorly controlled.

Air traffic controllers oversee today's busy airspace in hot, box-like towers which often resemble saunas. One of their biggest responsibilities is guiding small, private planes (referred to in the business as "kamikazes") among the big commercial jets that often use the same runways. Working at breakneck speed in order to prevent chaos in the skies, their clothes and chairs are often wringing wet at the end of their shifts. Controllers—and their families—suffer from a near-constant state of tension.[2]

Dr. Hans Selye made stress a household word when he described the "general adaptation syndrome" (GAS) as our pattern of response to extreme, unusual, or cumulative stressors. According to Selye, the body goes through several stages of adaptive response when confronted with a new source of stress.

The first stress response is the Alarm Reaction, in which the primordial instincts of the body prepare it to either advance or flee from an aggressor. If the body adapts to the source of stress, a period of resistance occurs where all the symptoms of the initial reaction disappear. However, Selye is quick to point out that if the source of stress is maintained, adaptation mechanisms eventually break down and a phase of exhaustion occurs. Symptoms of the initial alarm reaction reappear, but become irreversible. If these reactions are not controlled, the organism may die.[3]

The cumulative impact of cramped work space, temperature extremes, exposure to toxic fumes, and other stress factors may compromise the body's ability to cope with negative health factors. In commercial aviation, disaster may be the end result.

Common Signs and Symptoms of Stress ✈

You may experience some or all of the following symptoms after being exposed to a stressful environment: irritability, high blood pressure, anxiety, water retention, sensitive stomach, loss of a sense of humor, inexplicable moods, clouded thinking, insomnia, depression, nervousness, poor memory, fatigue, craving sweets, frequent colds, guilt feelings, constipation, diarrhea, lack of interest, alcohol/nicotine cravings.[4]

The Impact of Stress on Health ✈

The previously mentioned stressors for frequent fliers, aircraft personnel, flight controllers, and occasional air travelers are only part of the picture. Post-Traumatic Stress Syndrome is common among those who have been involved in any flying-related crisis. Symptoms include anger, mood swings, hallucinations, paranoia, nightmares, and guilt. Syndrome sufferers wonder why they were allowed to live while others died. They want to know what more they could have done to prevent death or injury among those around them. The phenomenon is similar to that noted among Vietnam War veterans whose lives were spared, but who witnessed the killing or suffering of their buddies.

Until a few years ago, there were no support groups to address these kinds of painful questions. Now there are many trained counselors and psychotherapists available who can help. Recognition of Post-Traumatic Stress Syndrome has led to the development of specific research programs and coping strategies for those enduring the aftershock of guilt or illness.

Stress and shock can manifest themselves long after the apparent conclusion of any crisis, including an aircraft disaster. Symptoms may be disguised as fatigue, illness, or debilitating neurosis. Human beings store memories of trauma even on a cellular level. Many health practitioners help their patients go through a process of "deep clearing."

There is evidence that airline crew members who have suffered the stress of bankruptcy, unexpected retirement, or working with incompatible crews can sometimes lose their sense of place and space. Such stressful circumstances are akin to a family enduring a complicated divorce, or losing a home in a disaster.

Practitioners treating people who have endured these situations report commonalties in such associated conditions as Chronic Fatigue Syndrome, Epstein Barr Disease, and allergic reactions. All are believed to be stress related and each can eventually break down the immune system.

Feelings of helplessness and the knowledge that there is no hope for restoring a work environment to its previous condition is heart breaking on many levels. A real fear sets in when people lose their financial and emotional stability as a result of industry-related stress.

Reactions to Stress ✈

Stressors exist both outside and inside the body. Low oxygen and humidity lead to anemia and dehydration, which become sources of physical strain that decrease one's ability to adapt to poor cabin air quality. A passenger's reaction is of key importance, and the nature of this response is contingent on the body's reserves. The healthier a person is physically and emotionally, the greater are his or her reserves for dealing with adversity.

People can usually cope with short-term stress, but frequent flyers and crew members experience multiple stressors at a greater frequency than most other people, as they are continually exposed to a hostile environment with little time for recovery. One flight attendant working international flights discussed the effects of stress frequent fliers often experience: "I noticed a big difference in personality. Not only in myself, but [in] those around me.

"[My coworkers and I] could not stand up under stress. We were snapping at each other. We were unable to do our work normally. I noticed my reflexes were completely off. I would be standing and then all of a sudden, just fall over or drop things. When I came home I would be so tired I would bump into walls and I would cry a lot. I just couldn't cope. "

Light and Stress ✈

The light conditions by which you work can stress both body and emotions. Cockpits, aircraft cabins, schools, and other indoor environments, which are either windowless or artificially illuminated, create ideal conditions for stress.

Continuous exposure to artificial fluorescent light may improve work performance for a short period, but productivity begins to decline over time. Such light sources are also believed to have adverse ionizing effects on the human body.

FAA Flight Surgeon James F. Crane has noted that, "in the artificial atmosphere of fluorescent light, all the spectral colors are not represented. The significance of this is a potential increase in stress reactions. Natural light fluctuates in brightness and color. Artificial light does not.

"In an aircraft, luminescence varies from the cockpit to the tail, depending on the time of day and the direction of the flight. The sun influences the psycho-physical efficiency of the body, but [when] fluorescent sources of energy [are used] the continuous exposure produces a stress reaction."[5] Note that aircraft interiors are primarily lit by fluorescent light.

Dr. John Ott, an expert on the effect of light on humans, believes everyone must have a "balanced diet" of natural, unobstructed sunlight absorbed directly through the eye. Artificial light does not duplicate the sun's rays, he points out. Glare shields, sunglasses, and tinted windshields also block sunlight.

Reducing Stress for Healthier Flying ✈

In order to overcome the negative health effects of stress, it is a good idea to take time out every day to partake in some stress reduction activity. Meditation, deep breathing, visualization, physical exercise, and laughter are all proven methods of mitigating the adverse physiological effects of stress. Some of these activities can be carried out frequently during the course of an airplane flight. Others, such as physical exercise, are great diversions and effective releases for the unvented reserves of "flight or fight" energy that abnormal amounts of stress can cause.

Each person has a set of individual strengths, weaknesses, and nutritional requirements. For this reason, I suggest you evaluate each of the following stress-reduction recommendations according to your own needs and temperament.

* *Listen to your own body.* People who lead ambitious, busy lives tend to ignore the silent signals their bodies are constantly sending out. Bodies have innate wisdom that is communicated to the mind and emotions, giving us the opportunity to make more intelligent choices. These silent signals may indicate injury or sickness. Take time occasionally to sit quietly and allow your body to get in touch with itself. At the same time, silently ask yourself questions about your health habits. Are you taking antacids, aspirin or alcohol to get through the day? If so, these are sure signs that you need to slow down and pay more attention to your physical being.

* *Moderation in all things.* The body loves change, yet it resists it. This is why gradual, moderate change is best, giving the body time to adjust to something new. Flight crews and frequent travelers make physical changes rapidly and often, which is a real test of adaptability. Do you know your own limits?

* *Ask for help.* Americans tend to suffer from the delusion that they have to do everything themselves without ever sharing their problems with others or asking for advice. This can be unhealthy. Talk to someone who has had experience with your problem.

* *Visualize health and relaxation.* It is helpful to prepare yourself mentally and emotionally for major changes through the use of the creative mind. For example, imagine yourself feeling good throughout a smooth and uneventful flight. Picture yourself unaffected by time zone changes. Tell your body that it can handle this trip easily

and even enjoy it. See yourself landing and deplaning, alert and refreshed, ready and eager for the next experience. This type of mental exercise (called "visualization") is frequently used by successful pilots and flight attendants. A similar exercise involves lying down and relaxing, as if in preparation for sleep. Breathe slowly and deeply. Mentally scan your body from head to toe. Imagine yourself looking from the outside in and from the inside out. Be on the lookout for areas where there may be pain, blockages, and so on. Observe yourself in detail, and wherever you sense a blockage or unwanted energy, visualize those elements flowing away from the body and dissolving into space.

♦ **Breathing and meditation.** Although it may sound absurd on the surface, it can be said that many of us do not know how to breathe correctly. People tend to take shallow breaths using only the top part of their lungs, rather than the entire abdomen. To exhale properly, draw in the abdominal muscles to push air out of the lungs. In order not to hyperventilate, you should breathe out slightly longer than you breathe in. The shoulders should not move up and down. Deep, slow breathing balances and centers the body's energy as it calms and relaxes. Rhythmic breathing can also be used to stimulate and energize. If you practice the following simple exercise, it will soon become automatic and natural. In a crisis, taking a few moments to breathe this way will make you ready for calm, centered action. First, inhale to the count of four or six, and then hold your breath in to the count of two or three. Finally, exhale to the count of eight.

You may increase the count to 8-4-16 or 16-8-32. Just remember to breathe out about twice as much as you breathe in to avoid hyperventilating and getting dizzy.

This is the beginning of meditation, a great stress reducer that has been used effectively for centuries. Many meditators have found that the longer they practice, the younger they look and feel. Research has shown that, through various kinds of breathing-related meditation, high blood pressure is reduced, hearing and vision are improved, and headaches recede.

One final tip from airline crew members: you can reduce the stress of jet-age travel by keeping a small bag packed with personal grooming items, such as a toothbrush, toothpaste, shampoo, makeup, a hairbrush, and any other items of choice. Have a list ready for other things you might need for a future trip. Use carryon luggage whenever possible.

Exercise, Relaxation, and Laughter ✈

Unless one has disc damage or other serious spinal ailments, there is nothing like yoga exercise, isometrics, and instructor-led aerobics to keep a body trim, supple, and relaxed. These movements can be performed easily in a confined space.

If nothing else, touch your toes several times a day, keeping knees straight. Turn your head left-to-right and right-to-left. Drop the chin to the chest, then tilt backward. Lift and drop the shoulders several times.

Do deep breathing before each exercise session. If bad weather or lack of space prevent walking or jogging, use a jump rope. Aerobic exercise videos and jump ropes take up very little luggage space. On the other hand, jogging in cities with highly concentrated air pollution is *not* recommended. Of course, you can also take advantage of a hotel swimming pool or sauna, or walk around any available gardens, parks, or grounds.

Laughter is one of the best tension relievers and is a great refresher. You can laugh in the privacy of your own room. Turn on the TV and watch a comedy instead of the evening news.

There has been much discussion about how the mind helps control stress and disease. Dr. David Spiegle, Dr. Herbert Benson, and the late author Norman Cousins appeared on ABC-TV's "Good Morning America" in April 1990, to talk about tests that revealed a rise in red corpuscle count during heightened emotion, and how other inappropriate body defenses are brought into play during stress. They emphasized the value of self-awareness, meditation, and breathing exercises as means of reducing stress and preventing disease.[6]

Chapter 12

INFLIGHT EMERGENCIES
AND PASSENGER SURVIVAL

The president of the Airline Safety and Health Association, Peter Trask, told the U.S. Senate Subcommittee on Aviation that people who fly assume that, "the price of their ticket takes care of enough fresh air, takes care of toxic fume protection, takes care of getting them out of the aircraft in case of any kind of problem. The ticket price should take care of that. I just think we are all being a little confused as to what the airlines are providing."

Peter Trask's conclusion that the flying public knows little or nothing about the actual circumstances aboard a commercial aircraft holds profound implications for the passenger. His or her ticket buys time for a seat in which life is—quite literally—at stake. Therefore, don't ticket purchasers have the right to know all of the conditions under which they make their decision to fly?

Education Means Survival ✈

Crew members and other expert witnesses appearing at Senate's aviation subcommittee hearings agreed that the airlines historically have wanted the public to know few details about the conditions in which they fly. For example, the consensus among speakers was that companies print only information their management has determined passengers "need to know" on the safety information cards available at every seat.

The FAA appears to support this attitude by focusing on the enforcement of issues arising within the organization itself, rather than from among the flying public or cabin and cockpit crews.

When Hawaii's Senator Daniel Inouye pursued this matter with Matthew Finucane, director of health and safety for the Association of Flight Attendants, Finucane declared flatly: "The FAA is an agency that really does not like ideas that are not invented at the FAA."[1]

With such disturbing comments at the bedrock of aviation industry governance, it is no wonder that selective information disseminated by regulatory agencies may be insufficient for an accurate understanding of the hazards that await consumers.

Meanwhile, airline deregulation and competition has reduced the number of flight attendants. Since flight attendants are specially trained to handle onboard emergencies, the implications are potentially life-threatening. The FAA requires at least one flight attendant for each fifty occupied seats, but "prior to the [economic] hemorrhaging of the airline industry, the number of flight attendants on a plane exceeded the minimum," according to Carol Austin, master executive council president for USAir's membership in the Association of Flight Attendants. Many carriers now use a "variable staffing" strategy whereby personnel are assigned according to the number of people booked. But if more passengers show up at the airport than were originally booked, no new staff can be assigned. "The lower numbers take a toll," says Austin, "both on fliers and those who serve them."[2]

How to Assess an Emergency ✈

It is entirely possible that you may be involved in an airline emergency some day. If this happens, will you be ready?

For instance, do you realize that there may be vastly different causes for some emergency situations that have the same outward manifestations? A sudden decompression such as that which occurred in the 1988 Aloha Airlines accident could be accompanied by a loud, ripping explosive sound, much like that of a bomb. Meanwhile, a rapid, *non*-explosive decompression might be followed by condensation that looks like smoke, but actually is not.

Guidelines for an appropriate passenger response:

* Grab your oxygen mask, pull the cord sharply, cover your nose and mouth, then breathe. (Do not use masks if smoke and fire is present since smoke can be drawn into it.)
* Make sure your seat belt is fastened, low and tight.
* Listen to crew commands
* Don't panic. Use common sense. Look around you and determine what, if anything, you can do to help. Remaining calm in your seat and following instructions may often be the best thing you can do.
* You should be familiar with all of the plane's emergency exits and the procedures necessary for either a ground or water landing. These details are quite different from one aircraft to another.[3]
* If your assigned exit is blocked by fire, water, or structural damage, change your course. Go to the next usable exit or deplane through a crack in the fuselage.

Safety Information ✈

Dr. H. Beau Altman and Dr. Daniel A. Johnson of the Interaction Research Corporation concluded that passenger inaction to an emergency situation ("negative panic") is just as common as the panic usually encountered in the aftermath of a disaster.

"When an emergency occurs," they point out, "those passengers who know what to do are less likely to exhibit maladaptive behavior than those non-educated to safety procedures. Training increases the probability of survival."[4]

After an Air Canada plane made a forced landing at Cincinnati in 1986, accident investigators found that many of the twenty-three passengers who died remained sitting in their seats, while survivors had memorized exit locations and managed to escape the smoking wreckage.

At one time the airline for which I flew showed passengers emergency procedure films before each takeoff of wide-bodied aircraft. Travelers were much more attentive than when the flight attendants demonstrated the procedures manually. The airline later discontinued the films on many of its domestic flights, citing prohibitive costs. In view of the poor response from passengers to the cheaper approach, I am convinced that reinstatement of visual demonstrations should be mandatory on all flights.

Considering the large number of flying-related hazards that have been proven by hard data, an information card should be made available on all flights informing passengers of the airborne pollutants, radiation, and other risks to health and safety that are present in the cabin.

The president of Interaction Research Corporation, a manufacturer of seat pocket safety cards, has written a book called *Just In Case*, which describes what to do in airplane emergencies. It is available by writing the author, Daniel Johnson, at his Olympia, Washington-based company.

All of these actions could be enforced by a federally mandated airline passengers' "Right to Know" Act.

Procedures for Safer and Easier Flying   ✈

When you board an airplane, do you look to see the number and location of safety exits on board? Are you aware that some overseas carriers block off exits over the wings in order to install extra seats for extra revenue? Ask your travel or airline agent if *all* emergency exits are available for use, especially those over-wing exits that may sometimes prove inaccessible.[5]

Although most passengers are probably unaware of them, the FAA has a set of minimum requirements that apply to all passengers sitting near emergency exits. A card explaining these standards should be in every seat pocket of the plane. Make sure the card is there, that you have read it, and that your flight crew has complied with its restrictions. The following guidelines are summarized from an exit row card and include specific restrictions that apply to occupants of such a seat. You must be able to:

- read English well enough to understand the instructions for opening the exits
- see well enough to observe signals given by crew members and such outside dangers as smoke or water (which would make the exit unusable)

- hear well enough to understand English commands
- speak well enough to give information to crew members or passengers during an emergency
- use all of your limbs, and be strong enough to open exit doors that weigh as much as sixty-five pounds
- help passengers get away from the plane
- and be at least 15 years of age and traveling with no one who requires your care

If you are unable to meet all of the above qualifications, you should not sit in an exit row. Ask the flight attendant for another seat if the exit row is assigned to you.

Also, it's always wise to find out what rights your carrier has to change, delete, or add to the terms of its ticket contract. Ask your travel or ticket agent for this information.[6]

Is Your Baby Safe? ✈

Attention was drawn to the air travel industry's lack of child safety seats during investigation of the 1991 Avianca crash on Long Island and the 1987 Sioux City, Iowa, United Airlines disaster when it became clear that many of the youngest passengers on these planes—babies and small children—were killed or injured.

In August, 1992, the *Wall Street Journal* described a course taught by former flight attendant Linda Pearson on how to survive an airplane disaster. She noted that unrestrained infants may become "deadly projectiles" during a crash.

This issue has been brought to the attention of both the airlines and the FAA for as long as children have been allowed to fly on commercial airlines. Flight attendants and concerned parents have made many appeals for child-restraining safety seats but have been met with avoidance and delay by those in a position to require such equipment.

As of October 15, 1992, air safety seats are permitted—but not required—for children under age two, provided they can be securely attached to a forward-facing passenger seat. Carriers charge for safety seats occupied by their infant passengers. Those younger than two now travel for free when seated on an adult's lap (where they are exempt from safety belt rules). In the case of a sudden stop or crash landing, having an unrestrained child on a passenger's lap has proven unsafe.

Some airlines will allow the use of an automobile safety seat on their flights, but it is wise to check with your travel agent and/or carrier to make sure such a device is allowed on the carrier you have chosen. Almost all of the auto safety seats manufactured after February 26, 1985, are acceptable for use on commercial aircraft.

(The FAA says some car safety seats manufactured between Jan. 1, 1981 and Feb. 25, 1985 are acceptable if they have either of the following labels: "This child restraint system conforms to all applicable federal motor vehicle safety standards," or, "This restraint is certified for use in motor vehicles and aircraft.")

You can obtain a free, detailed brochure on choosing and using child safety seats by sending a stamped, self-addressed envelope to: "Family Shopping Guide," American Academy of Pediatrics, 141 Northwest Point Blvd., P.O. Box 927, Elk Grove Village, IL 60009-0927.[7]

Protecting Your Baby in a Crash ✈

There is still some question as to whether the present air travel emergency procedures applied to infants and small children are truly effective. Above all, in an emergency, listen to instructions from members of your flight crew. They will advise you about how to brace yourself and your child. The following safety procedures generally apply to all aircraft:

FOR A LAP CHILD: Fasten your seatbelt securely around your body, not the child's. Hold the infant diagonally across your body with his or her head on the soft part of your shoulder. When instructed to "brace," lean forward with your head down.

FOR A SMALL CHILD IN HIS OR HER OWN SEAT: Make sure the child's seatbelt is securely fastened. If it is too loose, place padding such as pillows behind and under the child. You and/or another adult must sit in the seat next to the child. The child is to assume the "brace" position when told to do so. You are to assume your normal brace position, except only one arm will be placed behind your knees. The other arm is to be placed over your child with your hand on his or her neck. This keeps the head down and provides reassurance to the child.

Disabled Persons Are Not Guaranteed Access ✈

Although the "Americans with Disabilities Act" (which bars discrimination against the disabled in employment and provision of various services) became federal law in 1992, rules implementing the "Air Carrier Access Act" (which specifically bars discrimination against disabled persons by airlines) have not been issued by the Secretary of Transportation. This means that there is a stronger legal basis for airports to provide basic services to the disabled than airlines.

In an incident described in the December, 1992, *Condé Nast Traveler* magazine, a reader described how he had requested fully reclining seats in first-class in order to accommodate a child being sent to San Francisco for special spinal surgery. When the passenger checked in, the airline refused to accommodate the child, even after it was explained that she would be in severe pain if forced to fly in an upright position. A spokesman for the Department of Transportation, which enforces laws protecting disabled passengers, conceded that the airline was within its rights to refuse the request and was not obligated to offer compensation to the complaining party.

The bottom line is that if you need special assistance, access ramps, or a wheelchair, you should make sure ahead of time that there will be someone available who can help you. If you need special equipment aboard the aircraft, ask the airline in advance. If you want to bring your own equipment on aboard, representatives can tell you how you must stow it, or whether it will be allowed aboard the aircraft at all.[8]

Traveling Abroad ✈

Traveling in foreign countries may require some forethought on the part of today's traveler. Political unrest and street crime are widespread. Also, many countries have endemic or epidemic diseases for which a traveler may wish to receive vaccinations or other preventive medication.

The State Department has a Citizens Emergency Center, which offers free updated travel information and "consular information sheets" for every country in the world. These advise travelers of political unrest, diseases, earthquakes, volcanic eruptions, terrorism, and so on. The releases replaced the previous three-tiered "advisory" system of "warnings," "cautions," and "notices" at the end of 1992, and are not necessarily meant to discourage or bar a person from traveling to a particular country, but are designed to provide specific information that might not be available through the media.

Travelers may call the Citizen's Emergency Center at (202) 647-5225 to receive updated information. They may also find travel notices posted at thirteen regional passport agencies throughout the United States, the U.S. Customs service, and some travel agencies. Those considering a trip abroad can contact the Department of State's Bureau of Consular Affairs, Washington, D.C., 20520. Call (202) 647-5225 for an advisory.

For a free copy of *Precautions Abroad,* write: Overseas Citizens Service, Department of State, Room 4800, Washington, D.C., 20520. If you do find yourself in trouble when traveling abroad, U.S. embassies can help you, including keeping you advised of local disasters or political unrest as well as provide information on where to obtain food and shelter. Reports of airport closings and available flights will also be passed on.[9]

For complete information on traveling abroad, including advice pertaining to health, safety, and political unrest, write: Travel Medicine, Inc., 351 Pleasant St., Suite 312, Northhampton, MA, 01060, (413) 584-2670. You can also call your local Public Health Department or check with the consulate of the country you are visiting. Representatives of the airline on which you are traveling can sometimes give you necessary information about conditions in countries they serve. The Centers for Disease Control in Atlanta maintain an international travelers' hot line to answer questions about disease and vaccination. For information call (404) 332-4559 during business hours.

Chapter 13

HOW TO BE FIT FOR FLYING
THROUGH PROPER
NUTRITION

Sharon, a veteran flight attendant who had flown for about a dozen years, told me she recommends frequent fliers take vitamin supplements whenever they take a long trip. "I question whether or not the food on the airplane has nutritional value," Sharon said, emphasizing that "your body is put in extreme stress."

"I tried to eat properly," added Terry, another attendant, "but it was very difficult. When you are on an airplane for 12 hours you just eat when you can. It was not a proper diet and that is why, when I became pregnant, I felt it was very important not to fly....It is not a healthy environment for pregnancy."

The stress of airplane travel can be measured and evaluated in many ways. It includes meeting tight schedules, waiting in lines, carrying luggage, and putting up with crowded seating, poor air quality, and radiation exposure. Many people are sensitive to crowds, motion, and noise, adding yet more stress to their journey. All these demands substantially increase the body's energy requirement. Therefore, it is essential that flying crews and frequent flyers develop lifestyles that minimize the effects of additional stressors in order to maintain good health.

People with healthy habits—who exercise aerobically at least twenty to thirty minutes three times each week, eat nutritiously, and find ways of staying happy and satisfied—seem to better handle the vagaries of modern life.

Healthy Eating ✈

Statistics tell us a lot about our eating habits. For example, per capita consumption of soft drinks has risen 80 percent between 1945 and 1990 (the average soft drink contains eight to twelve teaspoons of sugar, or such artificial sweeteners as aspartame). Sales of pastries are up 70 percent, and potato chip sales are up 85 percent. Consumption of dairy products, meanwhile, has gone down 21 percent during the same period. Vegetable consumption is down 23 percent, and fruit purchases have plunged 25 percent.

There are over 2,000 additives in our food. These are chemicals used to color, flavor, preserve, and condition what we eat. Not only do these chemicals lack nutritional value, but they may be toxic as well. The average person eats three to five pounds of chemical additives and/or pesticides each year.[1] At the same time, most farm soil has become so depleted that our food does not contain the nutrients it once did and dietary supplements are often needed to avoid deficiencies.

"You are what you eat," is a popular adage, but nutritionists prefer to tell people, "You are what you assimilate." Eating the wrong food may poison some people, yet these same foods can be miracle cures for others. Milk can be a soothing, nourishing food for some, but in many cases it can cause intestinal upset, excess mucous formation, or allergic reactions.[2] Low-level lactose intolerance can mean gas and constipation after eating milk or ice cream (a problem when confined inside an airplane).

The connection between health and nutrition cannot be ignored or denied. As an accumulation of evidence and experience has shown, many of our major health problems can be relieved, prevented, or controlled through diet. For instance, the stress-related diseases of diabetes, heart disease, arthritis, asthma, ulcers, and cancer all have been successfully treated or ameliorated through careful manipulation of diet.[3]

Nutrition Basics ✈

Every statement you read or hear about food and nutrition comes from a particular bias based on the writer's (or speaker's) education, philosophy, cultural tradition, habits, gut feelings, and information received from friends and teachers.

Even the scientific community has not been entirely objective because its members have failed to examine their own personal and fundamental assumptions about health and nutrition. It is important to recognize such biases because only then can you judge whether the information is acceptable and useful to you.

Physician Ralph Luciani, nutrition counselor Phoebe Hummel, and I recommend a modified, natural-food diet as the best way to eat healthfully and to cope with stress. By "natural" we mean eating fresh food (in a form closest to its original plant or animal state) put through a minimum of processing. Unfortunately, optimal healthy foods are seldom found in restaurants, and the demands of career, family, and travel do not always allow for balanced or "natural" eating. For this reason, supplementing one's diet with vitamins, minerals, enzymes, and other nutrients is often necessary.

The Three Main Food Groups ✈

Foods are broken down into component parts: fats, carbohydrates, and proteins; which in turn contain vitamins, minerals, enzymes, and fiber. The first three components are also described in terms of their energy value (measured in calories). Simply counting the number of calories tells nothing about the *quality* of the food consumed. All calories are *not* alike.

Carbohydrates ✈

Carbohydrates are the body's main source of energy. They keep us warm and help regulate use of proteins and fats. Sugars, starches, and fiber are all carbohydrates. These are broken down into glucose—the body's energy source. Some glucose is used right away and some is stored as glycogen. Eating complex carbohydrates allows this process to occur slowly. But eating refined sugars causes the insulin-producing pancreas to overact, causing "reactive hypoglycemia" or low blood sugar.

Hypoglycemia (low blood sugar) and diabetes (high blood sugar) are two sides of a similar problem, both related to improper response to starches and sugars. Hypoglycemia can be due to an organic cause, but more frequently it is a reaction to stress or diet. Reactive hypoglycemia can be a result of the overproduction of insulin, underproduction of adrenal hormones, or liver dysfunction. The pituitary gland, which triggers many hormone releases, can also be involved.

Diet supplementation with vitamin C, niacinamide, vitamin B6, vitamin B12, pantothenic acid, and B complex generally help regulate carbohydrate metabolism. Also helpful are chromium, calcium, magnesium, potassium, and small amounts of sea salt.[4]

Proteins ✈

Proteins are the "building blocks" used in the growth and repair of all body tissues. They are made up of amino acids—some of which can be produced in adult bodies, but ten of which must be consumed in food. These "essential" or "indispensable" amino acids must be present at the same time and in the right proportion to one another in order to be used by the body as complete proteins. They are found in meat, dairy products, eggs, and fish, or can be combined from a mixture of certain plant foods.[5]

There is a great deal of controversy about the proper amount of protein needed and which source of protein is best. The National Research Council recommends that .42 grams of protein per pound of body weight be eaten daily. Your own protein requirements must be understood in relation to your specific metabolic type, your digestion, and the nature of your work. Around age forty, hydrochloric acid and pancreatic enzymes tend to diminish, and the proteins you eat will not be digested as well as they should be. This may cause bloating, gas, constipation, etc.

Proteins also may be broken down into carbohydrates for energy or storage. If proteins and carbohydrates are eaten together, the body will use the carbohydrates for energy and spare the proteins. A diet high in protein will force the body to utilize the protein for energy and mobilize the body's stored reserves of fat. This may be desirable for some people, high protein diets have been used in weight-loss programs. However, eating foods high in protein places added stress on digestive organs, especially the pancreas as well as kidneys. Many foods high in protein—especially meat and dairy—also contain high concentrations of fat.

Fats ✦

Saturated and unsaturated fats, and their impact on our health, are an important subject for research in the 1990's. Saturated fats, which are solid at room temperature, are strongly correlated to heart and arterial disease. Most saturated fats are of animal origin, except for cocoa butter, palm oil, and coconut oil. Unsaturated fats are liquid at room temperature and are mainly derived from seeds, grains, nuts, olives, or beans. Fish, especially those living in the cold water of the deep sea, contain omega-3 fats. These are very beneficial in producing increased levels of High Density Lipoproteins (HDL), which help offset the negative effects of high cholesterol.

Fats are not all bad. They provide energy, carry vitamins (A, D, E, K), support the inner organs, lubricate the skin, insulate the body and nerves, and are used to make hormones. However, the typical American diet is much too high in fat: it usually comprises about 40 to 45 percent of our total calorie intake. Even government health agencies and cancer research institutes recognize that this percentage is excessive. Too much fat not only contributes to obesity, but is deposited in the arteries and liver where it interferes with vital functions and causes life-threatening diseases. The "big three" non-AIDS-related causes of death (other than accidents) in the United States—cardiovascular disease, cancer, and diabetes—are all linked to excessive fat consumption.

An example of a low fat regimen is the Pritikin Diet, which allows only 5 to 10 percent fat, 10 to 15 percent protein, and 80 percent carbohydrates (vegetables, grains, beans).[6] This diet has proven to be successful in preventing repeat heart attacks and in managing many chronic diseases. The Pritikin approach—recently updated in *Beyond Pritikin* by Ann Louise Gittleman—provides a very good basis for eating, with one important exception. In accordance with the conviction that "whole food" is best, if your choose to eat eggs (preferably not exceeding four to six a week) I believe you should eat the entire egg, not simply the white. Consult your physician if you have a cholesterol problem.

The amount of fat recommended in the Pritikin Diet may be inadequate for cold weather climates, and intake amounts may need to be increased to 20 percent. During periods of hard physical work you might also need to increase your protein intake.

For details on supplements, check your local library or health food store. One of the best references I have found is the *Nutrition Almanac* edited by John D. Kirschmann.[7] Another book is *Prescription For Nutritional Healing*, by James Phyllis Balch.[8]

How to Maintain Good Health While Flying ✈

I began learning about proper nutrition in order to regain the good health I had lost after several years of flying. The changes in my diet were based on my own experience researching health and nutrition, as well as expert advice provided by Dr. Ralph Luciani and Phoebe Hummel. Working with them, I have developed twelve essential guidelines for life-affirming health habits. I offer them to you in the belief that they are the most important things one can do to maintain well-being while flying.

- Eat a protein meal (unless you have a protein allergy) at the beginning of your work day. At least drink a couple of tablespoons of protein powder added to milk or juice.
- Do not go more than six hours without food since this can cause low blood sugar. Carry a snack, but do not depend on sweets since protein helps prevent low blood sugar
- Do not depend on sugar or caffeine to get you up and going. The short-term energy boost they may provide can subsequently cause "rebound fatigue" and other hypoglycemic symptoms.
- Sip unsweetened fruit juice or lemon mineral water during a flight to reduce dehydration. Avoid drinking from the airplane's water supply as cleanliness and metal corrosion of the holding tanks is in question. Do not drink alcohol or soft drinks: they increase fluid loss.
- Do not diet while flying.
- A good diet should be based mainly on fresh vegetables. These can be either cooked or raw depending on one's

taste. Vegetables contain vitamins, minerals, and fiber, besides being low in fat. When eating in restaurants, choose dishes that contain the largest amount vegetables. Fresh fruit, whole grains, lean meat, fish or poultry, dairy products, beans, nuts, seeds, and beverages can either supplement or form the basis of a well-balanced meal.

◆ Avoid eating fried food. Your diet should contain a maximum of 20 percent fat, preferably less. Food saturated in fat or oil is much harder to digest and can make you feel bloated and lethargic.

◆ Do not allow yourself to become constipated. If necessary, take an herbal laxative after you arrive at your destination. Be familiar with your laxative so you will not be "surprised." Eating large amounts of grains (if you can digest them easily) and keeping well-hydrated usually helps prevent constipation. Dr. Jay Thomas, a colon therapist who has treated many flight attendants, reports that an impacted colon (due to dehydration and constipation) is a common ailment among flight crew members. You should have a minimum of one bowel movement a day.

◆ Be careful of your salt intake.

◆ Nutritional supplements (vitamins, minerals, glandulars, digestive enzymes, or special food concentrates) are recommended to offset the physical effects of any stressful condition. Stress places additional dietary nutritional requirements on any organism. If you smoke, or are exposed to smokers, you need extra vitamins A, C, and E. (If you have high blood pressure and/or heart problems, check with your physician about appropriate use of these vitamins.) For those susceptible to motion sickness, recent medical evidence suggests that the herb ginger (in capsules) is superior to Dramamine. (Ginger is not advised if a hemorrhoid condition exists.)

◆ Find a way to exercise at least five times a week for intervals of at least one-half hour each. On the airplane, move your legs to improve blood circulation.

◆ Pause a moment before digging in to your meal. Eating

too fast promotes gas and indigestion.

At best, eating what is available on plane flights or in airports may be unbalanced and inadequate to supply your body with the energy it needs to cope with the stress of flying. Therefore, it is wise to bring along such healthful foods as granola bars or trail mixes that are free of sugars, fats, and preservatives. Also, if your airplane is grounded for repairs or you are stranded at an airport, do not forget your continuing energy needs.[9]

Nutritional Therapy Tips ✈

Nutritional therapy encourages the use of dietary supplements (vitamins, minerals, amino acids, etc.) to help maintain optimum health when coping with today's modern food and lifestyles.

Recent studies demonstrate the benefits of such antioxidants[10] as beta carotene, Vitamin C, and Vitamin E. Use of these supplements is recommended for air travelers because they help keep the body healthy and boost its immune system. Research has isolated Vitamin E, in particular, as a possible preventative for heart disease, cancer, stroke, cataracts and dozens of other disorders.

Individual amino acids, which are protein building blocks that can affect neurotransmitters (the mechanisms that send messages between cells) are often used in nutritional therapy. This is an outgrowth of research into brain function at the cellular level, which has determined that neurotransmitters facilitate communication between brain and nervous system cells. For example, serotonin is a neurotransmitter that favors relaxation and sleep, whereas norepinephrine and acetylcholine stimulate activity.[11]

For Relaxation ✈

Instead of using alcohol or pharmaceuticals to help relax after a hectic flying schedule, try using natural substances. The "sleep vitamins" are vitamin C, B6, and inositol. Both vitamins C and B6 have anti-anxiety or sedative effects. The following nutrients are suggested sleep aids described by Dr. Carl Pfeiffer in his book *Mental and Elemental Nutrients*.[12] Check with your doctor before using sleep aids of any kind.

Calcium and magnesium—Suggested amounts: 500-2000 mg. calcium plus 400-800 mg. magnesium. A powdered or liquid form dissolved in hot water or milk is easily assimilated. Calcium taken with fruit juice or milk also helps absorption. These minerals are calming to both nerves and muscles. The traditional bedtime cup of hot milk contains both calcium and magnesium. Combining this with a cracker, cookie (whole grain, of course) or peanut butter sandwich, increases the positive effects. Calcium is especially helpful for cramps, whether menstrual cramps or leg cramps. Take one tablet every half hour for a total of 3 or 4 tablets.

Vitamin C—Suggested amounts: 500-3000 mg. Vitamin C may have an anti-anxiety or sedative effect when taken before sleep. If its acidity bothers you, take a buffered form. Equal amounts of bioflavanoids enhances absorption.

Inositol—Suggested amounts: 50-1000 mg. taken thirty minutes before bedtime. This is a B vitamin found in lecithin and cereals. It reduces stress-related high blood pressure.

Vitamin B6—Suggested amounts: 25-100 mg. This substance is needed in order for many enzyme reactions to occur, some involving brain and nervous system function.

Niacin/niacinamide—Suggested amounts: 50-400 mg. Niacin (a B vitamin) relaxes a person by dilating blood vessels and lowering blood pressure. This causes the characteristic "flush" of itching and red skin in niacin-sensitive people. Niacinamide, however, does not produce these effects and is not so directly beneficial for relaxation.

Single B vitamins—Should always be taken along with a B complex for balance. (It is believed that if one B vitamin is taken the liver stops producer other B vitamins.)

Herbs that are relaxing or sleep-promoting include chamomile (in the form of tea), hops, passion flower, skullcap, and lavender. A popular sedative herb is valerian, but since it is also habit forming, it is not recommended. Herbal formulas for sleep disorders can be purchased at health food stores. Herbal tea bags are easy to pack and take along on trips.

A hot bath can help you relax, especially if it contains one cup each of baking soda and sea salt, along with one quarter cup of hydrogen peroxide. Breathing exercises, meditation, and massage also promote relaxation. Biofeedback (a form of meditation induced by technology) can help one relax, as well as portable electronic "sound conditioners" which generate "white noise."

For Mental Alertness ✈

Instead of caffeine, try natural stimulants to stay alert.

Activity-inducing amino acids include phenylalanine (which also suppresses appetite), tyrosine (which can be converted into phenylalanine by the body), and glutamic acid (the nutritional form of which is L-glutamine). The non-sugar sweetener, aspartame, contains Phenylalanine, but is not recommended because it can raise one's blood pressure or cause severe headaches and insomnia, and must be strictly avoided by people with Phenylketonuria. Vitamins C and B6 metabolize Phenylalanine.

Other Applications ✈

L-glutamine—Along with glucose, L-glutamine is a brain fuel. This compound has been used to fight fatigue, depression, and impotence. It may also stop the craving for alcohol and sweets. Nutrition counselor Richard Passwater suggests doses of 500 mg. three times daily for a week or two, then decrease to two 500 mg. capsules twice a day.[13]

Choline—This B vitamin is used to form the acetylcholine necessary for memory, concentration, muscle coordination/response, and lubrication of mucous membranes. It is contained in cereals and lecithin. The effective dosage is 350-2000 mg. per day. Large doses of choline bitartrate (2000-3000 mg.) can cause diarrhea, so begin with small quantities and increase gradually. It tastes unpleasant, so have a fruit juice chaser ready. (Some people's bodies give off a fishy smell after taking choline chloride in large quantities.) Pantothenic acid is required for proper metabolism of choline (10 mg. of pantothenic acid per 100 mg. choline). Both choline and inositol are lipotrophics; that is, they aid fat digestion and reduce cholesterol.

Folic Acid—Folic acid functions as a coenzyme in the biosynthesis of norepinephrine and serotonin.

L-Phenylalanine—Used by many brain cells to stimulate each other, it is an extremely powerful anti-depressive nutrient.

Those with PKU (Phenylketonuria) must absolutely avoid it.
Ribonucleic Acid—This is an important natural substance for speeding up learning and aiding memory (known as RNA).
Potassium—Potassium is a necessary mineral that helps prevent nervousness, irritability, and mental disorientation.[14]
Vitamin A—Researchers believe supplemental amounts of this vitamin may stimulate the body's protective immunity response and help prevent certain types of cancer. It helps the liver in the detoxification process and, in the form of beta carotene, protects the body from internal and external stressors. Vitamin A deficiencies can lead to night blindness, dry skin, itchy eyes, and more serious problems.

In general, it appears that carbohydrates are converted into energy more readily in the morning, while they tend to be stored as fat in the afternoon. Fruit tends to be better utilized by the body in the morning, and vegetables are assimilated more effectively in the afternoon. Alcohol seems to have a stronger effect when one is rested rather than active. Aspirin is also more effective and lasts longer when one is inactive. Immune proteins, blood sugar, clotting time, heart rate, adrenal hormones, tolerance to pain, and numerous other processes vary throughout the day according to one's own individual circadian rhythms.[15]

Royal jelly, a glandular secretion made by worker bees, is rich in pantothenic acid, B vitamins, and essential amino acids. It includes a high concentration of lysine and such minerals as calcium, iron, potassium, silicon, and sulfur. Royal jelly is believed to be helpful in combating stress, fatigue and insomnia.[16]

Finally, homeopathic cell salts appear to be helpful in maintaining both cellular and overall health.[17]

A Nutritional Supplementation Model ✈

Dr. Ralph Luciani, Phoebe Hummel, and I endorse the following general daily vitamin consumption guidelines established by Dr. Jeffrey Bland, a renowned nutritional biochemist:[18] (Also recommended is *Diet and Nutrition* by Rudolph Ballentine.) vitamin A, 5000 i.u.; vitamin D3, 400 i.u.; vitamin E, 100 i.u.; vitamin C, 100-500 mg.; vitamin B1, 5 mg.; vitamin B2, 5 mg.; vitamin B3, 10 mg.; vitamin B6, 10 mg. (30 mg. for women using oral contraceptives); vitamin B12, 10 mg.; Pantothenic acid, 100 mg.; Choline, 100 mg.; Inositol, 100 mg.; Folic acid, 400 mcg.; PABA, 50 mg.; Calcium, 400-800 mg.; Magnesium, 200-400 mg.; Iron, 10-14 mg.; Chromium, 10-40 mcg.; elenium, 50-100 mg.; Manganese, 10-15 mg.; Copper, 1-3 mg.; and Zinc, 10-20 mg.

This type of formula can be found in a multiple vitamin/mineral supplement. In order to compensate for any kind of stressor, some of these nutrients may need to be multiplied two to ten times above the recommended minimum requirements, especially vitamin C. Therefore, one multi-vitamin pill taken daily would most likely be insufficient. When tailoring a program for your own specific needs you should consider taking a stress-type of B complex and a multiple mineral formula, as well as additional single nutrients or glandulars. You may prefer to take beta-carotene (instead of vitamin A and bioflavanoids) to enhance the action of your buffered vitamin C.

High quality supplements can be obtained from a health food store or nutritional physician. Some large groceries are also now carrying health food brands. Be advised that drug store and supermarket vitamins often contain sugar, yeast, fillers, and dyes that should be avoided. "Natural" vitamins are usually a combination of concentrated foods plus synthesized or extracted vitamins. When in doubt, read the labels. It is also important to get periodic blood-mineral analysis and to have a nutritional evaluation.

Cleansing and Detoxification ✈

Whatever you eat must be either digested and assimilated or eliminated. The process begins with chewing and the secretion of ptyalin, which starts the breakdown of starches into sugars. Protein digestion begins in the stomach where minerals are dissolved by hydrochloric acid. Pepsin, pancreatic enzymes, and bile continue the process in the small intestine. If any or all of these digestive enzymes are lacking, proper food digestion will be affected. The use of any of the digestive enzymes in supplement form will help correct the problem, along with dietary changes. A tincture of bitter herbs (such as Fernet Branca, which can be purchased in bars or liquor stores as "bitters") taken twenty to thirty minutes before eating stimulates digestive juice secretion. Drinking one teaspoon of vinegar in a glass of water after eating adds a small amount of helpful acid.

If you have ulcers, you may benefit from raw potatoes or deglycerrhizinated licorice as digestive aids. The latter is available in chewable tablets which also contain bismuth. It stimulates gastric mucous to protect the stomach lining. If gas is a problem, pancreatic enzymes can also be very helpful.

After a long period of eating irregular meals and airport, airplane, or restaurant food, detoxifying can give your digestive system a needed rest. (After all, you clean your house; so why shouldn't you clean out your body?) Along with your food it is likely you absorbed preservatives, toxic metals, and insecticides.

Constipation may occur because of irregular scheduling and dehydration. A diet low in fiber adds to the problem as the colon needs bulk in order to function normally. Taking acidophilus in yogurt, capsules, or liquid form helps normalize intestinal function by replacing "harmful" bacteria with "friendly" bacteria.

A colon cleanser made of ground-up or whole psyllium seed mixed with water or juice can be taken every morning, or whenever you get up. Its action is simply a result of adding bulk and will not "surprise" you. This morning routine can be expanded to a cleansing fast for one to three days by drinking one teaspoon of psyllium seed in juice, water, or broth four to six times a day. Drink plenty of water (six to ten glasses) during this period and take an herbal laxative the first day or two to "get things started." The fast can help remove toxins, rest the bowel, and also help clear the blood of symptoms from immune complexes.

Another very simple cleansing fast requires eating nothing but apples or watermelon seasoned with a squeeze of lemon or lime juice for two to three days. Drink plenty of water during this fast and take psyllium seed or an herbal laxative if necessary.

Low Blood Sugar ✈

The term "low blood sugar" (hypoglycemia) can be confusing. Even a person with normal glucose metabolism experiences low blood sugar if he or she has not eaten for six to eight hours. Low blood sugar can lead to mental and physical fatigue. People often eat high calorie snack foods such as chocolate bars, which stimulates the pancreas to secrete insulin at a faster rate. Unfortunately, this sudden jump in production is followed a short time later by a significant drop in insulin production, followed by the body's craving for still more sugar. Caffeine has a similar effect. This is why it is recommended that you take along your own protein sources when traveling, such as powdered drinks or wafers, nuts, oatmeal, and even granola bars.

Special Nutritional Needs of Frequent Fliers ✈

Frequent flyers must be especially mindful of proper nutrition. Consumption of proper nutrients is essential for the quick and efficient repair of stressed tissues, and for the maintenance of mental clarity and emotional balance. Depending solely on airplane food or fast food available at airports is a serious mistake.

At its best, the food served on airplanes is usually bland and over preserved, but passengers are likely to be so bored or hungry that they may often eat it anyway. I remember a pilot announcing a dinner entree selection of barbecued beef or teriyaki chicken. Then he added: "Don't worry if you don't get your first choice, because they both taste exactly the same."

Food Poisoning ✈

A study by Dr. Kenneth N. Beers and Dr. Stanley R. Mohler concluded that "gastrointestinal illnesses are the most common cause of inflight pilot incapacitation."[19] There have been many instances of passenger and flight crew illness resulting from the ingestion of contaminated airplane food. The meals are often cooked in ovens that are cleaned with toxic cleansers.

According to a 1992 article in the *Los Angeles Times*, seventy-six out of 336 people aboard a flight from South America to Los Angeles contracted cholera after being served tainted food. The illness eventually killed one passenger. Apparently the source of this infection was a seafood salad prepared in South America and distributed on board.[20]

For obvious reasons, the FAA has strict rules stating that all members of the cockpit crew cannot eat the same meal and that their meals must be prepared in separate kitchens. There are questions about how aggressively these regulations are enforced.

Food or water poisoning symptoms can include nausea and vomiting, intestinal cramping and diarrhea, chills and fever, and weakness and prostration. Obviously, food poisoning experienced during or after a flight can also be the result of eating local food.

Over-the-counter remedies such as Pepto-Bismol, Kaopectate, or Imodium may be helpful in relieving food or water poisoning symptoms. The homeopathic remedy known as Arsenicum Album is also excellent. If symptoms are severe and/or persistent one should see a doctor as soon as possible.

Replacement of fluids, vitamins, and electrolytes lost during bouts of diarrhea is essential. Electrolytes are the minerals potassium, magnesium, calcium, and sodium. Small packages of powdered electrolytes are available at health food stores and in the pharmacies of many developing countries. Tomato or fruit juice can also help replace electrolytes.

Advice from the Flight Crew ✈

What do pilots and flight attendants think of the meals served on the airlines they fly? Some shared revealing thoughts with me.

Sharon said she took extra vitamins whenever she flew, and also grew vegetables for home-cooked meals. "If you don't have proper nutrition in your diet you mentally and physically become very run down," she explained. "You are dealing with numerous viruses because of the many people you encounter, and your body needs a bigger defense. You must take vitamins."

Sonja also took vitamin supplements. When asked her opinion of airplane food, Sonja said she was "concerned about the preservatives in it," adding that she preferred to take her own food on board. She recalled reading an article in *Time Magazine* estimating it took five to ten days for airplane food to work through the body before it is completely flushed out.

Natural Cosmetics ✈

The following are beauty tips tested by flight personnel in airplane cabins and other dry, stressful environments.

Cucumbers and lemons are great complexion aids. After

cleansing the face, splash with diluted lemon juice and water in order to create a good acid-alkaline balance, then seal and tighten pores by rubbing the skin with a slice of cucumber. A scrub made with cold cream and table salt is also effective. For very dry skin, it might be best to use an oily cleanser rather than soap. Chamomile tea bags can be put in the refrigerator after use and placed on your eyes the morning after you return from a trip. The liquid soothes and clears the eyes and shrinks the puffy bags underneath them. A raw, shredded potato will do the same trick.

Ear, nose and throat specialist Dr. Arthur L. Schiller recommends using salt water or the saline product *Ocean* to keep sinuses open and moist in the dry air cabin environment.

Wheat germ oil is a great conditioner for face and hair. It may discolor blonde hair, however, so blondes are better off using mayonnaise. An avocado mashed with wheat germ oil and egg yolk serves as a complete meal for skin and hair. The body absorbs nutrition from the outside as well as the inside. The effects are immediate and leave a healthy glow. Fresh strawberries mashed together with butter and applied to the face rejuvenates the skin. Patting honey on the face provides the skin with nutrients and stimulation, which firms the skin and tightens pores.

For those with oily skin, egg whites and aloe vera gel both make for good facial masks. A clay mask applied once a week tightens the skin, removes dead cells, and improves circulation. Avoid applying the mask to the tender skin under the eyes; the skin will be drawn downward and dried out too much. Pat a moisturizer under makeup and keep applying it during a flight.

My favorite nighttime facial applications are sweet almond oil and Beleza Original Protein, which can be ordered through Sanfi Corporation Beauty Products, 850 N. Cypress St., Orange, CA, 92667. During the day I use Epicurean Enzyme Skin Nutrition, available through Epicurean Enzyme, 26081 Via Viento, Mission Viejo, CA 92691. A nice body massage oil can be made out of a combination of peanut oil, olive oil, lanolin, and vitamin E. Avoid mineral oil (a petroleum product) because it may destroy vitamin E, which is essential to healthy skin.

Chapter 14

WHAT IS—AND ISN'T—BEING DONE TO MAKE FLYING SAFER AND HEALTHIER

The Federal Aviation Administration has proven to be a major stumbling block in ongoing efforts to improve conditions for those who fly. Despite the fact that it is the government agency primarily responsible for air traveler safety, the FAA has often denied the need to add major protective provisions to its regulations. In fact, as many as twenty years may pass before action is taken on a matter of pressing importance, at which time the agency happily takes full credit.

During the early 1980s, the National Research Council first recommended a ban on all smoking aboard U.S. commercial aircraft. The first step toward that goal was a prohibition on smoking involving flights of two hours or less. Bills addressing a complete ban were presented to Congress on October 7, 1987, and adopted in 1988. The ban took effect February 25, 1990. However, smoking is still allowed on most international flights (except those of Air Canada, Northwest Airlines, and Quantas).

The U.S. Congress is not exempt from criticism in any discussion of air travel safety, as a small but revealing incident suggests. In 1988 the Senate killed a measure (previously passed by the House) that would have required that a toll-free consumer "hotline" telephone number to the FAA be printed on the bottom of all airline tickets.[1]

Another illustration of the FAA's lackluster performance was the revelation in late 1993 by independent investigators that the agency's own planes were flying without benefit of the same basic safety programs it expects airlines to follow. The National Transportation Safety Board said the fatal October 1993, crash of an FAA plane may have been affected by the fact that the pilot took off without an instrument flight plan (despite bad weather), he and other pilots had no training to help them work with copilots (standard procedure among commercial airlines), and there is no surveillance to ensure the safety of FAA flight operations. An FAA official said the agency accepted the NTSB's criticisms and was addressing them.[2]

The Chaos of Deregulation ✈

Paul Stephen Dempsey, a director of transportation law and author of *Flying Blind: The Failure of Airline Deregulation*, believes that what began "as a program of modest liberalization became an avalanche of abdication of responsible government oversight. . . . Deregulation has been associated with unprecedented levels of [economic] concentration, discriminatory pricing, service deterioration and narrower safety margins." By 1989, according to Dempsey, consumers were paying 2.6 percent more to fly per mile than if the pre-deregulation downward trend in pricing had been allowed to continue.

Earlene L. Causey, CEO of the American Society of Travel Agents, told *USA Today* that specialized taxes and fees collected from airlines should be used "to improve the air traffic control systems and airport infrastructure. There should be financial incentives to encourage rapid investment in technologies that will improve customer service, reduce airline costs and raise consumer satisfaction." In the same article, USAir CEO Seth Schofield agreed that "carriers must do better at managing their assets."[3]

Airline labor groups have certainly felt the impact of deregulation, and not in a positive way. "Although new entrants enjoyed significantly lower labor costs in the inaugural years of deregulation," Dempsey observes, "the squeeze on carrier profits unleashed by deregulation has forced management to exact serious concessions in terms of labor wages and work rules." In *Flying Blind*, Dempsey offers a legislative reform proposal, "which attempts to steer a common sense course between heavy-handed regulation and laissez faire." His hope is that comparisons between what was promised and what has been delivered by deregulation will give future decision-makers thoughtful pause.[4]

Quick settlement of a five-day 1993 strike against American Airlines by 95 percent of its flight attendants showed labor's rebounding strength after twelve years of industry deregulation under the Bush and Reagan administrations. Staffers overturned management's attempt to trim the number of attendants per flight and cut salaries. President Bill Clinton intervened in the strike after American's chief executive officer rejected arbitration.[5]

Aging Aircraft ✈

Hearings on the subject of aging commercial aircraft were held between 1986 and 1989 by committees of both the U.S. Senate and House, but no initiatives were forthcoming. Roger Fleming, senior vice-president for technical services of the Air Transport Association, has maintained that the problems surrounding aging aircraft have been exaggerated and are not a serious safety issue. However, Representative Guy Molinari (R-NY), an FAA critic and member of the House Public Works and Transportation Committee, believes that the hazards posed by aging aircraft have been both minimized and overlooked.[6]

In 1991, the Aging Aircraft Safety Act was enacted, requiring an FAA rulemaking that would mandate inspections of airliners with fifteen or more years of service "to ensure continuing airworthiness." The new law provides for training of FAA inspectors and engineers related to corrosion and metal fatigue.

Safety Inspectors and Inspections ✈

The Aviation Subcommittee, chaired by Rep. Norman Mineta (D-CA), held hearings in 1983 on the validity of the Reagan administration's 25 percent cutback and convinced then Transportation Secretary Elizabeth Dole to reinstate positions that were eliminated. This was partially accomplished in 1984, but the Bush administration subsequently delayed spending for aviation programs once again, apparently due to funding the 1990 Gulf War.

"Simply adding more inspectors is not the total answer," Rep. Paul Hammerschmidt (D-AR) emphasized at the hearings. "Preliminary GAO findings indicate the problems extend beyond mere numbers. . . . Frequency of inspections among airlines varied from a high of eighty-six per 1,000 operating hours for one carrier to a low of one per 1,000 for another." In short, the GAO criticizes inspection methods and lack of follow-up.

The FAA still maintains that there are not enough inspectors to check all the planes; therefore it will not fine airlines which "appear" to be correcting safety problems. However, in recent years, the FAA has had to share the blame with McDonnell Douglas and General Electric for the faulty part which caused the 1989 crash of a United Airlines DC-10 in Sioux City, Iowa.[7]

In 1993, FAA official Anthony Broderick confirmed that, "because of budgetary constraints, [the agency] will not increase safety inspector staffing."[8]

Empty Control Towers ✈

The need for funds extends to all areas of aviation. The National Transportation Safety Board (NTSB) needs more investigators and the flight control towers have not been fully staffed since the debilitating PATCO (controllers' union) strike of 1981.

The General Accounting Office, in a statement before the congressional hearings on the status of the U.S. Air Traffic Control System, asserted that "1988 perceptions of the air traffic work force show little change since our 1985 survey."

Rep. Glenn M. Anderson (D-CA), chairman of the House Subcommittee on Investigations and Oversight, was disturbed to learn that in a single year, from 1988 to 1989, the FAA lost the services of some 150 air traffic controllers. "That says something about the system," Anderson mused.

Shifting priorities and budget cuts during the Bush administration put air traffic control staffing on hold. Hearings on pilot and air traffic controller issues are ongoing.[9]

Jim Burnett, chairman of the NTSB in 1987, claimed that his organization did not have the staff capacity to evaluate properly the latest flight control technology and that the FAA needs to be more sophisticated in its technical analysis. The GAO reported in 1987 that the advanced automation system and other labor-saving and efficiency increasing technologies that the FAA planned to incorporate were already eight to nine years behind schedule and not likely to be installed until the 1990s. The FAA confirmed in 1993 that full implementation of the Advanced Automation System program was still at least two years away.[10]

Cabin Air Quality ✈

Major health and safety problems related to cabin air quality were introduced in U.S. Senate hearings in 1981 and debated for the next seven years, then left dangling after the Department of Transportation recommended that the issue needed further study. In 1988, Hawaii's Senator Daniel Inouye once again presented language to cover the issue as part of S. 2367, The Aviation Research Bill. Inouye argued that it should be "within the mandate of the Civil Aeromedical Institute to develop research programs to evaluate and monitor environmental quality in airplane cabins for the protection and survival of aircraft occupants." The proposed legislation was still pending in early 1994.[11]

Radiation ✈

In 1967, an FAA advisory committee looking into cosmic radiation and its effect on airplane crew members reported that annual radiation doses were, "on the average, higher than those incurred in almost any other industry." Researchers found that those working on the high-altitude SST aircraft "may receive more than the five hundred millirems per year above the maximum permitted members of the general public." The advisory committee indicated that "it might be necessary to designate SST crews as occupationally exposed persons. In this case they will have to be informed of their exposure."

The FAA panel was disbanded in 1969 when the U.S. abandoned its short-lived SST program and consideration of inflight radiation exposure was not addressed again until 1984. Health physicist Edward T. Bramlitt then proposed a rulemaking that would formally classify flight crews as radiation workers within

the Federal Air Regulations. The FAA denied Bramlitt's petition
in March of 1986. Finally, in 1990, the FAA stated that it was in
the process of developing a new radiation advisory for crew
members. However, as of early 1994, it still had not been made
available to them.[12] In January 1993 pilots on some airlines began
to wear and monitor high altitude radiation detectors (dosimeters)
as a result of government advisement. Shortly thereafter, the
FAA acknowledged the cancer risk for crew and passengers flying a large number of miles and advocated "careful scheduling of
personnel to avoid persistent exposure to higher radiation levels
associated with high altitude flights and flight paths crossing extreme northern and southern latitudes." Still, no official protocol
has been established for dosimeter use.[13]

Collision Avoidance ✈

In a report to the House Committee on Public Works, Rep.
Glenn Anderson (D-CA) complained that technology, which
could make routing of airplanes safer (referred to as the Traffic
Alert and Collision Avoidance System (TCAS)), had suffered un-
derdevelopment since the 1950s.

It was not until the end of 1987, Anderson pointed out, that
the Airport and Airway Safety and Capacity Expansion Act was
enacted. Its provisions required that TCAS be installed on all
commercial aircraft of at least thirty seats. A final ruling affirm-
ing this requirement was issued in early 1989. By 1993, 80 percent of the 54,000 aircraft subject to this order had been equipped
with TCAS, according to the FAA.[14]

The airline industry, claiming that the compliance schedule
would not allow enough time for proper maintenance and engineering changes, asked for an extension. So, in an effort to satisfy both interests, Rep. Ron Packard (R-CA) amended the TCAS
implementation schedule to require 25 percent installation by December 30, 1990, 50 percent by the close of the following year,
with completion by the end of 1993.

The Packard bill allowed a one-year extension to the current
100 percent installation deadline, and the FAA later confirmed
that the schedule would not be met until 1994. In addition, the bill
allowed the FAA Administrator to extend the December 30,

1991, 50 percent installation deadline. The bill also called for the FAA Administrator to consider adjusting the current wind shear installation schedule to match that which was proposed for TCAS. (The current wind shear detection equipment installation schedule called for 50 percent implementation by January 2, 1991 and 100 percent after two more years.) As of February 1993, only 106 major airports had installed the equipment.[15]

The FAA has speculated that, had the upgraded TCAS been on board the airline aircraft involved in several midair collisions (including four California disasters that killed 251 people), these accidents would have been prevented. However, despite a dramatic rise also in near collision reports, the FAA has delayed TCAS installation until 1997. This is also despite 1990 testimony before Congress by FAA Associate Administrator Anthony J. Broderick that implementation was "going very well."[16]

Infant and Child Safety Seats ✈

The issues regarding safety belts and special seats designed to protect infants and children have long been debated in commercial aviation. Legislation mandating such restraints was introduced in the House in July 1990, and is still pending. A proposed rulemaking on a child safety seat requirement is awaiting action by the FAA (along with initiatives involving fire extinguishers, protective breathing equipment, pilot training, collision avoidance, and wind shear). A regulation that went into effect on October 15, 1992, permitted—but did not require—the use of child safety seats in commercial aircraft. Carriers are allowed to charge full price for these seats, even when occupied by children under age two (who otherwise fly for free).

Anti-Terrorism and Air Piracy ✈

The escalation of terrorist acts aimed at commercial air carriers has prompted a new focus on aviation security. Joint hearings on the impact of international terrorism on travel were held before Congress in 1986. During those sessions, the U.S. State Department claimed that "in the brief time that the Anti-terrorism Assistance program has been in existence, it has become a valuable and effective tool in improving international cooperation to combat terrorism."

In 1993, the FAA's Anthony Broderick confirmed that twenty-eight of the forty-seven actions mandated in the Aviation Security Improvement Act of 1990 had been completed, including placement of additional security liaison officers overseas.[17]

However, when the Senate Committee on Foreign Relations asked H. Wayne Berens, president of Revere Travel and a member-at-large of the Travelers Security Policy Council, if the government's travel advisory procedures were adequate, Berens demurred. "I am not sure they are timely or adequate," Berens said. "Travel advisories are not needed 'after the fact.' Perhaps two levels of advisories are needed for earthquakes and other [natural] disasters, and a third for security related matters." Berens concluded by asking: "Is there perhaps too much scrutiny of information prior to the release of an advisory?"

Detection of Plastic Explosives   ✈

In 1982, officials of the U.S. government and the airline industry acknowledged that security measures to protect U.S. airliners abroad were inadequate and that organic materials such as plastic bombs could easily pass through existing detection systems. The FAA responded by expediting its order of six Thermal Neutron Analysis devices, that can effectively detect plastic explosives. It is unclear, however, why the FAA and airline companies did not make interim use of sophisticated new detection machines, such as the Three-Dimensional Intelligent Space system, which could also screen for plastics. As this book went to press, the FAA had tested Thermal Neutron Analysis devices at several airports and was evaluating further use of these and other alternatives.

Congressional legislation introduced to help solve this detection problem is still pending. As this book went to press, several crucial U.S. airports still had no equipment to detect plastic explosives or similar materials.[18] A second bill died at the end of the 1992 Congressional session.[19]

Another solution may lie in the use of explosive-proof cargo containers, tested successfully in England.

Conclusion

It is clear from a host of reliable sources—Senate and House testimony, research by health physicist Edward Bramlitt, statements by aviation industry officials, union safety files, and press reports—that commercial air travel poses many significant health and safety hazards to flight crews, frequent fliers, and the general population. I feel that the public will need to be made more fully aware of these serious problems before any meaningful change will come to the airline industry, the Federal Aviation Administration, and other regulatory agencies. Congress and the media have begun to investigate and address these complex problems, but those who fly are often oblivious to the ongoing debate about aviation health and safety risks and their potential solutions.

In summing up, I feel the greatest hazards for flight crews and the flying public, the ones which frighten me the most, are the lack of good quality control related to airplane safety (involving fleet fatigue and bogus parts) and the apparent lack of concern on the part of most airline and regulatory officials for cabin air quality, high altitude radiation, and passenger or crew health. These issues have widespread implications for the American public. Remember, over 300 million people fly each year, many of them regularly, and more than 100,000 flight attendants and crew members are exposed daily to the hazardous conditions aboard a commercial aircraft.

What Factors Contribute to Safety Hazards? ✈

The factor which contributes most heavily to these problems is stress. If cockpit crews, air traffic controllers, or airplanes themselves are suffering from too much stress, the problem cannot be ameliorated by simply pulling the plane over to the curb and stopping until the pressures go away.

Another important factor is illness. You may be flying with sick crew members whose judgment is impaired. And if the crew is flying without a contract and/or union protection after a bank-ruptcy reorganization, employees probably do not have sick leave or health insurance and thus often feel they must work even when not feeling well.

Why Are Airlines Neglecting Health and Safety? ✈

Why have these problems been allowed to occur in the first place? Airlines, especially after deregulation, are placing their highest priority on the *cost* of operations, often to the neglect of the safety and health of the people most closely involved in oper-ating their planes.

Admittedly, overhead costs would increase if airlines took the steps necessary to improve conditions for their passengers and employees. In my view, the most important of these include up-grading their aircraft, not accepting the cheapest (and perhaps bo-gus) spare part, giving radiation dose information to flight crews, cleaning up the cabin air environment, paying crew members an adequate living wage, making sure that flight attendants aren't overstressed by the hours they are working, and providing the latter with adequate emergency medical training enabling them to use all of the equipment in cabin first aid kits (rather than hoping a medic or physician will be on board).

The current laissez faire attitude obviously is not working. But trying to skimp on safety is not always the cheapest way to operate. If more and more aging planes blow their tops or drop into the ocean, if flight crews start demonstrating increased rates of cancer or other serious disease from the conditions of flying, liability costs will skyrocket.

Of course, cost is not the only factor involved: lives, liveli-hoods, and personal health are at stake. Remember, those cheap tickets may very well reflect cost-cutting by the airline that nega-tively affects maintenance, health, safety, and staffing.

Flying Isn't Fun Anymore ✈

How many people actually *enjoy* flying these days? I can remem-ber when flying was a real treat. Passengers once were carried smoothly across the skies—with beautiful vistas below—in clean, modern planes which could boast attentive crews, plenty of room to move, and good food.

Today, even as you are boarding a plane, you can start to sense the unpleasant experiences that lie ahead. Old equipment can mean blocked toilets, and you may be greeted by the smell of chemicals and smoke from days gone by. You are literally crammed into seats with little room for arms or legs. You sit through delay after delay on the ground, often breathing in toxic engine fumes in a stuffy, hot, and overcrowded plan.

Once in the air, you may have to crawl over three people whenever you wish to leave your seat. Flight attendants are often understaffed and too busy to attend to your special needs. The food usually tastes bland and preserved, the produce is not fresh, and part of the meal may even be even unrecognizable. The cabin can turn very cold and all the blankets will have been passed out. You may feel overwhelmed: by the roaring sound of the engines, the overcrowding, or the lack of cushioning in your seat and under the carpets (especally on newer planes).

You may arrive on the ground an hour or more later than expected due to delays in take-off and thus have to scramble for new connections, often running at full speed through an airport with luggage in tow (risking a coronary in the process). You may not even be able to find your luggage, especially if you missed a connecting flight.

How Will the Skies Become Safe? ✈

When someone finally wins legal redress because he or she contracted cancer due to years of being exposed to radiation in flight, the airlines will begin to listen. When consumers refuse to fly with an airline they feel is unsafe or doesn't attend to their health-related needs, airlines will start to implement changes.

If you care about safety conditions in flight, contact your representatives in Congress. Call the Department of Transportation, which estimates that less than two out of every 100,000 air travel passengers file a complaint each year (by the way, their consumer affairs office number is 202-366-2220). Write to the FAA and the airlines. Contact the Aviation Consumer Project at Public Citizen in Washington at (202) 833-3000. *Do something!*

Glossary

Agencies and Organizations

ACAP - Aviation Consumer Action Project
AFA - Association of Flight Attendants
AMA - Aerospace Medical Association or American Medical Association
ALPA - Air Line Pilots Association
ATA - Air Transport Association
ATC - Air Traffic Controller
ASRS - Aviation Safety Reporting System
cfpm - cubic feet per minute
CHRC - Citizens Health Research Committee
DOT - Department of Transportation
EPA - Environmental Protection Agency
FAA - Federal Aviation Administration
FAR - Federal Air Regulation(s)
FDA - Federal Drug Administration
FPC - Full Performance Controller
GAO - General Accounting Office
NASA - National Aeronautics and Space Administration
NATCA - National Air Traffic Controllers Association
NRC - Nuclear Regulatory Commission
NTSB - National Transportation Safety Board
OSHA - Occupational Safety and Health Administration
ppm - parts per million
TCAS - traffic alert and collision avoidance system
UFA - Union of Flight Attendants

Endnotes

CHAPTER 1 - Flying Low to Flying High ✈

1. B. Wade, "Keeping Fit In Economy Class," *New York Times,* Sunday, March 1989.
2. Anthony J. Broderick, Associate Administrator for Regulation and Certification, Federal Aviation Administration; letter to Rep. Bill Richardson (D-NM) in response to author's query; February 18, 1993.
3. *Condé Nast Traveler,* October 1992, pg. 160.
4. Peter S. Greenberg, "Survey Says: Alaska Airlines Rates Best Overall," *Los Angeles Times,* June 30, 1991; Christopher Reynolds, "Report on Airline Safety," Los Angeles Times, October 24, 1993, pg. L2.
5. *Collier's Encyclopedia,* P.F. Collier & Sons Corp., Vol. 1, 1966, pp. 369-372, 384-388, Vol. 3, 1966, pp. 372-377; Whitehouse, *The Sky's The Limit,* (New York: Macmillan, 1971), pp. 13, 14; "Airliner Cabin Safety and Health Standards," Hearing before the Subcommittee on Aviation of the Committee on Commerce, Science, and Transportation, U.S. Senate, 97th Congress, 2nd Session on S. 1770, May 20, 1982, (Washington, D.C.: U.S. Government Printing Office, 1982), hereafter referred to as S. 1770, Cabin Air Quality.
6. Edward T. Bramlitt, Ph.D., letters to NAS committee (and to author, 1986.
7. S. 1770, Cabin Air Quality, op. cit.; "The Airliner Cabin Environment—Air Quality and Safety," National Academy of Science (NAS) Committee on Airliner Cabin Air Quality, Board of Environmental Studies and Toxicology, Commission on Life Sciences, National Research Council, (Washington, D.C.: National Academy Press, August 1986), hereafter referred to as NAS Report.
8. Author's conversation with FAA information officer Phil Akers, March 1990.

CHAPTER 2 - How Flying Affects Your Lungs, Heart, and Other Vital Organs ✈

1. S. 1770, Cabin Air Quality, op. cit., pp. 24, 48, 70, 71, 90-92, 127; Hearing on Senate Bill S. 197 (formerly Bill S. 1770), September 19, 1986, p. 30. This bill later became Public Law 98-466, hereafter referred to as S. 197;

Edward T. Bramlitt, Ph.D., "Commercial Aviation Crew Member Radiation Doses," *Health Physics,* Vol. 49, No. 5, (November) 1985, pp. 945-948.

2. S. 1770, Cabin Air Quality, op. cit., May 20, 1982, pp. 35, 73, 144, 152.

3. Norva Achenbaugh, Chairperson, Health & Safety Committee, Association of Flight Attendants (AFA), statement, S. 197, p. 74.

4. Dan Rather News Special, CBS-TV News, March 1984.

5. Author's interview with anonymous flight attendant.

6. CBS Evening News with Dan Rather, CBS-TV News, June 9, 1993.

7. Author's interviews with flight crews, 1983-1990, op. cit., S. 1770, Cabin Air Quality, op. cit., pp. 24, 48, 70, 71, 86, 90-92, 127, 138, 163; NAS Report, op. cit., p. 3; Smoking Ban HR 2040, op. cit., p. 125.; Hearing on Senate Bill S. 197 (formerly S. 1770), September 19, 1986, p. 30. This Bill later became Public Law 98-466, hereafter referred to as S. 197; Edward T. Bramlitt, Ph.D., "Commercial Aviation Crew Member Radiation Doses," op. cit.

8. Letter to author from Bertil Werjefelt, President of Vision Safe Inc., and Founding Director of the Airline Safety and Health Assn. (ASHA), December 6, 1983; S. 1770, Cabin Air Quality, op. cit., Werjefelt statement, 1982, pp. 68-126; S. 1770, Cabin Air Quality, op. cit., p. 127.

9. NAS Report, op. cit., pp. 8, 167.

10. Anonymous flight attendant report to author; Andy Yates, retired captain, statement before the ASMA members, 1987.

11. "Committee Reports," *Union Update,* published by Airline Flight Attendants Assn. (AFA), November/December 1986, pp. 2, 9-10.

12. *Seattle Times,* May 1990.

13. NAS Report, op. cit., p. 120; *New York Times* interview with Rob Coppock, Board on Environmental Studies and Toxicology—JH 653, National Academy of Sciences, April 26, 1987, p. 25.

14. *New York Times,* June 5, 1993.

15. Letter from Anthony Broderick to Rep. Bill Richardson, op. cit.

16. Werjefelt letter to author, op. cit.; S. 1770, Cabin Air Quality, op. cit., pp. 128, 129, 133.

17. S. 1770, Cabin Air Quality, op. cit., pp. 70, 71, 126, 127, 133, 147-150; NAS Report, op. cit., pp. 48-50; Smoking Ban HR 2040, op. cit., p. 335.

18. S. 1770, Cabin Air Quality, op. cit., p. 127; Author's interviews with cockpit crews, 1983-1990, op. cit.; Author's conversation with Captain Benton Stephenson, former Eastern Airlines Senior Check Airman; Author's phone conversation with FAA representative, February 1990, anonymous.

19. S. 1770, Cabin Air Quality, op. cit., pp. 152, 153; Author's interviews with cockpit crews, 1983-1990, op. cit.; Author's conversation with Pat Wright, PAA Chief Pilot, January 21, 1984; Smoking Ban HR 2040, op. cit., p.335; NAS Report, op. cit., p. 32; Author's conversation with Captain Benton Stephenson, 1990; Federal Air Regulations (FARs), Section 121.

20. S. 1770, Cabin Air Quality, op. cit., pp. 71, 138-140; Werjefelt letter to author, December 6, 1983, op. cit.; Senate Bill S. 197, op. cit., statement from Peter Trask, pp. 105, 106.

21. NAS Report, op. cit., pp. 3, 4; Author's interviews with flight crews, 1983-1990, op. cit.; S. 1770, Cabin Air Quality, op. cit., pp. 152, 153; Senate Bill S. 197, previously S. 1770, Public Law 98-466, op. cit., p. 34.

22. S. 1770, Cabin Air Quality, op. cit., p. 47; Arthur C. Guyton, *Textbook of Medical Physiology,* Fourth Ed., (Philadelphia: W.B. Saunders, 1971), pp. 520-521; Weylin G. Eng, "Survey on Eye Comfort in Aircraft: 1. Flight Attendants," *Aviation, Space and Environ. Med.,* April 1979, p. 403.

23. "Medical Aspects of Transportation Aboard Commercial Aircraft," AMA Commission on Air Medical Services: Air Transportation, *Journal of the American Medical Association (JAMA),* February 19, 1982, Vol. 247, No. 7, p. 1009.

24. S. 1770, Cabin Air Quality, op. cit., p. 162; NAS Report, op. cit., p. 17.

25. S. 1770, Cabin Air Quality, op. cit., p. 48; NAS Report, op. cit.; Smoking Ban H.R. 2040, op. cit., pp. 123, 124, 125, 128. S. 197, p. 74.

26. S. 1770, Cabin Air Quality, op. cit., pp. 48, 49; "Committee Report," Union of Flight Attendants Local #1 (UFA), Health and Safety files, no date, p. 6; NAS Report, op. cit., pp. 17, 19, 165, 166; Arthur Guyton, *Textbook of Medical Physiology,* op. cit., pp. 520, 521.

27. "Committee Report," Union of Flight Attendants Local #1, op. cit., p 6.

28. NAS Report, op. cit., pp. 18, 167, 168; S. 1770, Cabin Air Quality, op. cit., pp. 144, 145, 146.

29. Arthur C.. Guyton, *Textbook of Medical Physiology,* op. cit.; "Cures for Common Complaints," *Travel & Leisure Magazine,* October 1987, p. 19; *The Merck Manual of Diagnosis and Therapy,* 13th Ed., (Rahway, NJ: Merck, Sharp & Dohme Research Laboratories, 1977), Div. of Merck & Co., Inc., p. 1206; NAS Report, op. cit., pp. 3, 4, 18, 167, 168.

30. "Cures For Common Complaints," *Travel & Leisure,* October 1986, p. 24.

31. S. 1770, Cabin Air Quality, op. cit., p. 145.

32. NAS Report, op. cit.

33. Ibid., p. 168.

34. S. 1770, Cabin Air Quality, op. cit., p. 152; John Poppy, "Air Travail," *Esquire,* September 1989, pp. 141-143.

35. NAS Report, op. cit., p. 165.

36. "Medical Aspects of Transportation Aboard Commercial Aircraft," op. cit., p. 1010.

37. Michael N. Emmerman, "Flying and Diving, Spring 1989 Update, The Investigation Continues," pp. 1, 2.

38. Arthur C. Guyton, *Textbook of Medical Physiology,* op. cit.; Dwight Dedmon, "Physiological and Psychological Deficiencies of the Airline Flight Attendant Induced by Employment Environment," op. cit.

39. NAS Report, op. cit., p. 166; C. Richard Wolf, M.D., "Aerotitis in Air Travel," UFA Committee Report, Berkeley, November, 1977.

40. "Occupational Health Guideline For Ozone," Occupational Safety and Health Administration (OSHA), September 1978, p.1; S. 1770, Cabin Air

Quality, op. cit., p. 90; Judith Goetz, *Jet Stress,* (Huntington Beach, CA: International Institute of Natural Health Science, Inc., 1980), pp. 19, 20.

41. C.E. Melton, "Effects of Long-Term Exposure to Low Levels of Ozone: A Review," *Aviat. Space Environ. Med.,* February 1982, p. 110.

42. Lisa Yates, Director of Health & Safety, Independent Union of Flight Attendants (IUFA), statement made before the Subcommittee on Aviation of the Senate Committee on Commerce, Science, and Transportation, S. 197 (Previously S. 1770, Cabin Air Quality), November 9, 1983, pp. 2, 3, 4, hereafter referred to as S. 197; Author's phone conversation with Lisa Yates, 1983.

43. Judy Goetz, *Jet Stress,* 1982, p. 19; Lisa Yates, "Statement for Hearing on Bill S. 197," op. cit., pp. 3, 4, 6-9; S. 1770, Cabin Air Quality, op. cit., pp. 48, 49, 88, 90; NAS Report, op. cit., pp. 5, 59, 113, 114.

44. "Occupational Health Guideline for Ozone," National Institute for Occupational Safety and Health (NIOSH), U.S. Dept. of Labor, September 1978, p. 1.

45. CBS Morning News, July 16, 1986, interview with Dr. David Hawkins, of the National Resources Defense Council and Carmen Gage, retired flight attendant; Linda Hamlin, "Ozone," one page article, available from author, source unknown; Lisa Yates' statement, op. cit.; C.E. Melton, "Effects of Long-Term Exposure to Low Levels of Ozone: A Review," *Aviation, Space and Environmental Medicine,* Vol. 53, No. 2, February 1982, pp. 105, 110; NAS Report, op. cit., pp. 116, 118, 193; S. 1770, Cabin Air Quality, op. cit., pp. 1, 48, 49.

46. C.E. Melton, "Effects of Long-Term Exposure to Low Levels of Ozone: A Review," op. cit.; S. 1770, Cabin Air Quality, op. cit., p. 67; Lisa Yates' statement, op. cit.

47. C.E. Melton, op. cit., p. 105; NAS Report, op. cit., pp. 51, 118, 119.

48. Federal Air Regulations, 121.578, New Code, 1985.

49. NAS Report, op. cit.

50. NAS Report, op. cit., pp. 15, 118, 193, 218; Lisa Yates' statement, op. cit., C.E. Melton, op. cit., p. 110; S. 1770, Cabin Air Quality, op. cit., pp. 21, 43, 67, 74; "Airliner Cabin Environment: Contaminant Measurements, Health Risks, and Mitigation Options," Report No. DOT-P-1589-5, GEOMET Technologies, Inc, 20251 Century Blvd., Germantown, MD, 20874-1192, December, 1989, p. 8-31.

51. Anthony Broderick letter to Rep. Bill Richardson, op. cit.; Federal Air Regulations, 25.832, New Code, 1985.

52. S. 1770, Cabin Air Quality, op. cit., pp. 45, 48-50; *Collier's Encyclopedia,* (Canada: P.F. Collier & Son Ltd., 1966), p. 204.

53. "Clearing the Air About Ion Machines," *Changing Times,* Vol. 34, December 1980, pp. 33-36; Albert Krueger, "Are Negative Ions Good For You?", *New Scientist,* June 14, 1973, pp. 668-670; Charles Wallach, "Ions and Your Health," Natural Air Quality Systems, 1979; Marian C. Diamond, "Uppers and Downers in the Air," *Psychology Today,* June 1980, p. 128.

54. Albert Krueger, "Are Negative Ions Good For You?," *New Science,* June 14, 1973, pp. 668-670.

55. Author's conversations with Phoebe Hummel, nutrition counselor, 1983-1990; C. McDonald Denmark, "Statement Before the Subcommittee on

Aviation of the Committee on Commerce, Science, and Transportation," U.S. Senate, Re: Senate Bill S. 197 (formerly S. 1770), 98th Congress, "Airline Cabin Safety and Health Standards," November 9, 1983; S. 1770, Cabin Air Quality, op. cit., p. 140.

56. Michael N. Emmerman, "Flying and Diving," op. cit., p. 3; B. Wade, "Keeping Fit In Economy Class," op. cit.

57. Michael N. Emmerman, "Flying and Diving," op. cit.

58. Daniel K. Inouye, Senator, Hawaii, "Press Release: Aircraft Air Study Proposal," November 9, 1983, p. 30; NAS Report, op. cit., pp. 2-4, 32, 33, 48-50; S. 1770 Cabin Air Quality, op. cit., p. 140; "Medical Aspects of Transportation Aboard Commerial Aircraft," op. cit., pp. 1007-1011.

59. S. 1770, Cabin Air Quality, op. cit., p. 73.

60. NAS Report, op. cit., pp. 8-167.

61. "Medical Aspects of Transportation Aboard Commercial Aircraft," op. cit., pp. 1007-1011; Dwight Dedmon, Health & Safety Officer, AFA, "Physiological and Psychological Deficiencies of the Airline Flight Attendant Induced by Employment Environment," *AFA Report*, September 30, 1968, p. 8; Arthur G. Guyton, *Textbook of Medical Physiology*, op. cit., pp. 520, 521; NAS Report, op. cit., pp. 118, 207, 208; Aerospace Medical Association, Committee on Medical Criteria, "Medical criteria for passenger flying, "*Arch. Environ. Health*, 2:124-138, 1961.

CHAPTER 3 - AIRBORNE BACTERIA, VIRUSES, AND DISEASE ✈

1. Elliot Dick, Ph.D., letter to author, 1986; Author's personal flight experiences and interviews with flight crews. Author's personal interviews with passengers, and crew reports.

2. S. 1770, Cabin Air Quality, op. cit., pp. 92, 118, 119; John Poppy, "Air Travail," *Esquire*, September 1989, pp. 141-143; Michael N. Emmerman, "Flying and Diving, Spring 1989 Update, The Investigation Continues," op. cit.

3. S. 1770, Cabin Air Quality, op. cit., pp. 25, 125, 134, 135, 154; NAS Report, op. cit., pp. 157, 162.

4. Bill S. 197, op. cit., pp. 30, 31.

5. S. 1770, Cabin Air Quality, op. cit., pp. 70, 71, 82-87, 92, 152-153; NAS Report, op. cit., pp. 152, 155-158; "Transmission of Rhinovirus Colds by Self-Inoculation," *The New England Journal of Medicine*, Vol. 288, No. 26, 1973, pp. 1362-1365; Letter from Elliot Dick, op. cit.

6. S. 1770, Cabin Air Quality, op. cit., pp. 70-71, 82-87, 92.

7. Dwight Dedmon, "Physiological and Psychological Deficiencies of the Airline Flight Attendant Induced by the Employment Environment," op. cit., pp. 8-9; Weylin G. Eng, "Survey on Eye Comfort in Aircraft: 1. Flight Attendants," op. cit., pp. 401-404.

8. NAS Report, op. cit., pp. 201, 202.

9. S. 1770, Cabin Air Quality, op. cit., p. 70.

10. Bertil Werjefelt letter to author, 1983, op. cit., p. 2; S. 1770, Cabin Air Quality, op. cit., pp. 10-13, 18, 19, 24, 25, 28, 29, 76, 77, 134, 135.

11. S. 1770, Cabin Air Quality, op. cit., pp. 77, 140; NAS Report, op. cit., pp. 159-160; "Aircraft Humidification," Aerospace Information Report, Air 1609, Society of Automotive Engineers, Inc., pp. 4, 30, 89.

12. Author's personal flight experiences and conversation with flight attendants, anonymous.

13. Rhonda Richards and John DuBois, "Outsmarting the Flu Bug," *USA Today,* January 18, 1994, pg. 5B.

14. Crew reports, 1983-1990, anonymous.

15. *The Merck Manual of Diagnosis and Therapy,* 13th Ed., op. cit., pp. 4, 76, 111, 507, 611, 1013, 1017, 1366, 1427, 1432, 1576-1577; NAS Report, op. cit., p. 152; "Transmission of Rhinovirus Colds by Self-Inoculation," op. cit., pp. 1361-1364; Author's phone conversation with hospital and immigration nurses, anonymous.

16. Author's phone conversation with Captain Bill Price, 1987.

17. Author's personal flight experiences and crew reports, 1967-1990; NAS Report, op. cit., pp. 153, 154, 162.

18. Elliot Dick, Ph.D., letters to author, 1990 and 1993; Dr. Silvio Finkelstein, "Who Whispers in Modern Cockpits?", *Air Line Pilot,* July 1989, pp. 16-17.

19. *Travel Indonesia,* January 1993, p. 24, and December 1992, p. 12.

20. Anonymous reports from flight attendants and cleaning crews.

CHAPTER 4 - Radiation in Flight ✈

1. The author is indebted to *Understanding In-Flight Radiation,* by Robert J. Barish, Ph.D., Research Associate Professor of Radiology, N.Y.U. Medical Center, published by In-Flight Radiation Protection Services, Inc., NY, April 1989, and to Edward T. Bramlitt, Ph.D., whose research has provided for much of the substance of this discussion.

2. W. Friedberg, Ph.D., D.M. Faulkner, M.S., L. Snyder, E.B. Darden Jr., Ph.D. and K. O'Brien, "Galactic Cosmic Radiation Exposure and Associated Health Risks for Air Carrier Crewmembers," *Aviation, Space, and Environmental Medicine,* November 1989, p. 1106.

3. Donald D. Engen, *Report to Congress, Airline Cabin Air Quality,* U.S. Department of Transportation, February 27, 1987, p. 15.

4. Keith Easthouse, "LANL scientist: Acid Canyon may have hotspots," *The Santa Fe New Mexican,* April 15, 1992, p. B1; Matthew L. Wald, "New Estimates Increase Radiation Risk in Flight," *The New York Times National,* February 19, 1990. p. A11. All statistics quoted in this paragraph derive from this article.

5. Niren L. Nagda, Roy C. Fortmann, Michael D. Koontz, Scott R. Baker, Michael E. Ginevan, "Airliner Cabin Environment: Containment Measures, Health Risks, and Mitigation Options," report No. DOT-P-1589-5, U.S. Dept. of Transportation, December 1989, prepared by GEOMET Technologies, Inc., op. cit.

6. Interviews with Jana Harkrider, Health and Safety Chairman, Flight Attendants (UFA), Local #1, Continental Airlines, 1983-1989; Andy Yates,

Chairman, panel on "Reproductive Functions of Female Flight Attendants," May
13, 1987, panelists included the author and the following people: Edward T.
Bramlitt, Ph.D., Albuquerque, NM, Stanley R. Mohler, M.D., Wright State
Univ., Kenneth Lyon Jones, M.D., Univ. of Cal. Medical Center, San Diego,
CA, Pamela J. Boltinghouse-Haines, R.N. (nurse-flight attendant), Sacramento,
CA; testimony from Matthew Finucane, Director of Safety and Health, Assoc. of
Flight Attendants (AFA), hearing on Senate Bill S. 197, Public Law 98-466, September 19, 1986, pp. 6-8; see Senate testimony, S. 1770, Cabin Air Quality, op.
cit., from Bertil Werjefelt, Director, Aviation Safety and Health Association, and
President, Vision Safe Inc., pp. 6-8; Matthew Wald, "New Estimates Increase
Radiation Risk in Flight," op. cit.

7. Anthony Broderick letter to Rep. Bill Richardson, op. cit.; Department of
Transportation report, Radiation Exposure of Aircrews and Recommended Limits, 1992.

8. Edward T. Bramlitt, Ph.D., "Reproductive Functions of Female Flight
Attendants," op. cit.; See "Radiation Protection Guidance to Federal Agencies for
Occupational Exposure," U.S. Environmental Protection Agency (EPA), Office
of Radiation Programs, Washington, D.C., 20460; see also Federal Register,
Vol. 52, No. 17, January 27, 1987, Presidential Documents, pp. 2822-34.

9. Edward T. Bramlitt, Ph.D., "Reproductive Functions of Female Flight
Attendants," op. cit.

10. W. Friedberg, et. al., op. cit., pp. 1104-1108.

11. Robert R. McMeekin, M.D., Radiation Exposure of Air Carrier Crewmembers, FAA Advisory Circular 120-XX, draft, undated. The most recent reference in this document points to September 1988, allowing me to speculate that it
was written in late 1988 or even 1989. Curiously, Friedberg, et. al. do not cite
McMeekin's work even though they use the same data base.

12. W. Frideberg, et. al., op. cit., p. 1106.

13. Matthew L. Wald, "Radiation Exposure is Termed a Big Risk for Airplane Crews," New York Times, February 19, 1990. p. A16.; Matthew L. Wald,
"Test of Cockpit Radiation Show Levels Above A Federal Standards," New York
Times, March 1, 1990, p. A22.

14. John W. Gofman, Radiation Induced Cancer from Low Dose Exposure:
An Independent Analysis, 1990, available from the Committee for Nuclear Responsibility, Inc., P.O. Box 11207, San Francisco, CA, 94101; Science, Vol.
247, January 5, 1990; Aaron Sugarman, "Radiation risk for pregnant fliers,"
Condé Nast Traveler, August 1990, pp. 29-30; Conversation between author and
Gofman, 1990; John W. Goffman, M.D., Radiation and Human Health, (San
Francisco: Sierra Books, 1982).

15. Kirby A. Van Horn, Captain, B-727, Continental Airlines, letter to the
FAA, re: Rules Docket AGC-204, August 28, 1989. Van Horn is responding to
Circular 120-XX.

16. Matthew Finucane, letter to FAA, Docket AGC-204, August 28, 1989.
He is also responding to FAA Circular 120-XX.

17. Robert J. Barish, Ph.D., Understanding In-Flight Radiation, op. cit.,
pp. 42-43.

18. Richard B. Stone, Executive Chairman for Aeromedical Resources,

Airline Pilots Association, August 19, 1989, letter to the FAA, Rules Docket AGC-204. He, too is responding to FAA Circular 120-XX; Robert R. McMeekin, M.D., *Radiation Exposure of Air Carrier Crewmembers*, op. cit.
19. Robert J. Barish, Ph.D., letter to FAA, Docket AGC-204, August 9, 1989.
20. Edward T. Bramlitt, Ph.D., Health Physicist/Chemist, panelist at Aerospace Medical Association (ASMA) meeting, May 13, 1987, "Reproductive Functions of Female Flight Attendants," op. cit., Audio Transcripts, 610 Madison St., Alexandria, VA 22314.
21. Author's phone conversation with Cay Pylate, 1987; David H. Wood, D.V.M., Ph.D., Michael G. Vochmowit, M.P.H., Ph.D., Yolanda L. Saimon, B.S., M.A., Robert Eason, D.V.M., and Richard A. Boster, D.V.M., Ph.D., "Proton Irradiation and Endometriosis," *Aviation, Space, and Environmental Medicine*, August 1983, p. 721; H.M. McClure, J.H. Ridley, and C.E. Graham, "Disseminated endometriosis in a rhesus monkey (Macaca mulatta)," *J. Med. Assoc. Ga*, 60, 1971, pp. 11-13.
22. Aaron Sugarman, "Radiation risk for pregnant fliers," *Condé Nast Traveler*, August 1990, pg. 29.
23. John W. Gofman, M.D., *Radiation and Human Health*, op. cit.
24. W. Friedberg, et. al., op. cit., pp. 1104-1108.
25. Richard A. Passwater, Ph.D., *Selenium as Food and Medicine*, (New Canaan, CT: Keats Publishing, 1980), pp. 216-225; See also "Low Selenium Levels and Cancer," *Aviation Medical Bulletin*, March, 1984, p. 3; William A. Ellis, "Antioxidant Enzymes: Protect Your Family Against Radiation," *Health Express*, Vol. 3, No. 3, April 1982, pp. 11-13; Stephen A. Levine, Ph.D. and Jeffrey H. Reinhardt, Ph.D., "Biochemical Pathology Initiated by Free Radicals, Oxidant Chemicals and Therapeutic Drugs," *Journal of Orthomolecular Psychiatry*, Vol. 14, No. 1.
26. Ingrid Naiman, Ph.D., "Radiation Exposure," *Welcome to Planet Earth*, Aquarius (February) issue, 1988, published by Mark Lerner; Frances Nixon, *Born To Be Magnetic*, Vol. 1, 1971, Vol. 2, 1973, (Victoria, BC: Magnetic Publishers); Serge King, *Earth Energies: A Quest for the Hidden Power of the Planet*, (Wheaton, IL: Quest Books, 1992).
27. Robyn Seydel, "Diet for a Small (Irradiated) Planet," *Earth Island Journal*, Winter 1988-89, Avery Publishing Group, p. 12.
28. Sara Shannon, "Diet for the Atomic Age," from *Earth Island Journal*, August 1987, Avery Publishing Group.
29. Robyn Seydel, "Diet for a Small (Irradiated) Planet," op. cit.
30. Robert O. Becker, M.D.; *Cross Currents*.

CHAPTER 5 - Emergencies On Board ✈

1. S. 1770, Cabin Air Quality, op. cit., pp. 8-9, 14-15, 35-42, 94-97.
2. Ibid., pp. 36-39, 95, 116-117.
3. S. 1770, Cabin Air Quality, op. cit; "Flight Attendants and Passengers Partners in Aviation Safety," *Passenger Safety Quarterly*, AFA, 1625 Massachusetts Ave. N.W., Washington, D.C. 20036, Vol. 1, No. 1, Summer 1989.

4. FAR (Federal Air Regulations) Amendment to 121.309.
5. S. 1770, Cabin Air Quality, op. cit., pp. 22, 23, 62; NAS Report, op. cit., pp. 9, 10.
6. Greg Wiles, *Honolulu Advertiser,* April 21, 1993, p. C-3.
7. NAS Report, op. cit., pp. 92, 101-103; Author's phone conversation with C.O. Miller, May 1990.
8. S. 1770, Cabin Air Quality, op. cit., pp. 62-63, 72-73, 141; episode of *Geraldo Rivera* syndicated television show; April 6, 1990.
9. NAS Report, op. cit., pp. 10-11.

CHAPTER 6 - TOBACCO SMOKE AND OTHER HAZARDOUS CARGO ✈

1. S. 1770, Cabin Air Quality, op. cit., p. 102; Author's interviews with pilots; Hearing to Ban Smoking on Airline Aircraft, Subcommittee on Aviation of the Committee on Public Works and Transportation, House of Representatives, 1st Session, October 7, 1987, pp. 35, 120, 124, 125, 128, 134, 135, hereafter referred to as Smoking Ban H.R. 2040; "Committee Reports," *Union Update,* op. cit. pp. 2, 9-10.
2. Smoking Ban H.R. 2040, op. cit.
3. Author's interview with anonymous flight pilot; Smoking Ban H.R. 2040, op. cit.
4. S. 1770, Cabin Air Quality, op. cit., p. 152; *Union Update,* op. cit., p. 2; NAS Report, op. cit., p. 295.
5. *New York Times,* interview with Rob Coppock, op. cit., p. 25; Smoking Ban HR 2040, op. cit., pp. 46-58, 71, 119-135; "Medical Aspects of Transportation Aboard Commercial Aircraft," op. cit.; M.E. Mattson, Ph.D., et. al., "Passive Smoking on Commercial Airline Flights," *JAMA,* Febuary 10, 1989, Vol. 281, No. 6, p. 867.
6. S. 1770, Cabin Air Quality, op. cit., p. 162; Stephen A. Levine and Parris M. Kidd, "Antioxidant: A Unified Disease Theory," *J. Orthomolecular Psychology,* Vol 14, No. 1, pp. 19-24; *Collier's Year Book, 1990,* p. 322; various Environmental Protection Agency studies, U.S. Government Printing Office, Washington, DC.
7. Smoking Ban HR 2040, op. cit., p. 121.
8. Letter from Mr. & Mrs. Buselli to Senator John Danforth, Chairman of the Senate Committee on Commerce, Science and Transportation, September 24, 1986.
9. Smoking Ban HR 2040, op. cit., pp. 93-94.
10. Ibid., pp. 128-129.
11. Ibid., pp. 124, 152.
12. Martin Tolchin, "U.S. Initiates Effort to Halt Spraying," *New York Times,* January 17, 1994; Linda Bonvie and Bill Bonvie, "Flying in the Mist," *Earth Journal,* November/December 1993, pp. 38-73.
13. NAS Report, op. cit., pp. 169-171; Author's conversations with flight and cabin cleaning crews.
14. Department of Transportation Airline Cabin Environment report, op.

cit.

15. "Pilots Signal Air Safety Problems, ALPA Applies Remedies," *Air Line Pilot,* May 1989, p. 47; Christopher Winans, "Risky Materials Often Find Way Onto Airplanes," *The Wall Street Journal,* November 21, 1989, B1, B5.

16. Anthony Broderick letter to Rep. Bill Richardson, op. cit.

17. Comment by Tim J. Vanden Heuvel to the FAA Docket No. 25959, "Air Line Pilots Association (ALPA) Petition for Rulemaking on Toxic Fluids," December, 1989; NIOSH ALERT, Request for Assistance in "Preventing Death from Excessive Exposure to Chlorofluorcarbon 113 (CFC-113)," May 1989; Special Bulletin, "Fluorocarbon 113...DON'T BE CAUGHT...DEAD!", Michigan Dept. of Public Health; Jan W. Steenblik, Technical Editor, TECHTALK, "ALPA Petitions FAA on Toxic Aircraft System," *Air Line Pilot,* August 1989, pp. 48-49.

18. Irene Jackson, *The San Diego Union,* Sept. 5, 1990, pp. B1, B5.

CHAPTER 7 - Fatigue, Flying, and Even Dying ✈

1. *Collier's Year Book,* 1990; Jan W. Steenblik, "Reducing Pilot Error: Who Will Take the Lead?", *Air Line Pilot, Journal of the Air Line Pilots Association,* Vol. 57, No. 2, February 1988, pp. 12-13.

2. Michael J. Weiss interview with former pilot John Nance, "In His Own Words," *People Weekly,* March 31, 1986; Robert C. Maynard, "Deregulated Skies: Book a Window Seat to See Free Market," *Albuquerque Journal,* September 4, 1986, p. A5; "Year of the Near Miss," *Newsweek,* July 27, 1987, pp. 20-27, SIRS, Vol. 3, Article No. 53, pp. 1-4; "More Facilities Needed to Avoid Gridlock in Air," *Atlanta Journal and Construction,* August 2, 1987, pp. C1+, SIRS, Vol. 3, Article No. 54, pp. 1-6; "Where are the Controllers?", *Richmond Times-Dispatch,* August 9, 1987, pp. F1+, SIRS, Vol. 3, Article No. 56, pp. 1-4; "The Black Box," *Air & Space,* June/July 1988, pp. 31+, SIRS, Vol. 3, Article No. 72, pp. 1-4; Aviation Safety (Near Midair Collisions and Runway Incursions), Hearing before the Subcommittee on Investigations and Oversight of the Comm. on Public Works and Transportation, House of Representatives, 100th Congress, First Session, April 9, 1987, U.S. Govt. Printing Office, Wash., D.C., 1988, pp. 2, 4, hereafter referred to as Collisions and Incursions; Gordon Witkin, "Wanted: A Dozen New Airports," *U.S. News & World Report,* January 25, 1988, pp. 32-33; SIRS, Vol. 3, Article No. 63.

3. AFP and Reuters press dispatches, April 1993.

4. "Year of the Near Miss," *Newsweek,* op. cit., p. 2; Richard Witkin, "FAA Says Delta Had Poor Policies on Crew Training," *New York Times,* September 19, 1987, pp. A1, A11.

5. "In His Own Words," *People Weekly,* op. cit., pp. 93, 94; John Nance, *Blind Trust,* William Morrow & Co., New York, 1986.

6. Letter and report to author from Vincent J. Mellone, Deputy Program Manager, Aviation Safety Reporting System (ASRS), February 7, 1990.

7. "Year of the Near Miss," op.cit., p. 2; Collisions and Incursions, op. cit., pp. 2-3.

8. *USA Today,* December 30, 1993.

9. "In His Own Words," *People Weekly,* op. cit., pp. 93, 94; Charles A. Jaffe, "Wind Shear," *St. Petersburg Times,* March 9, 1986, pp. A1+, SIRS, Vol. 3, Article No. 27.

10. Veronica L. Young, Producer-Director, "Why Planes Crash," NOVA series, PBS television network, January 20, 1990; Michael Specter, "The FAA's Sweat Shops," *Washington Post,* January 5, 1987, National Weekly Edition, pp. 6-7, SIRS, Vol. 3, Article No. 41, p. 2.

11. Martin Tolchin, "F.A.A. Finds More Errors by Air Traffic Controllers," *New York Times,* January 1, 1994.

12. Statement by Richard L. Stone, coordinator for the Human Performance Project, to the Air Line Pilots Assn. (ALPA), July 1983; C.V Glines, "New Rules for Old Issues," *Air Line Pilot,* November 1985, pp. 25-30; "In His Own Words," *People Weekly,* op. cit., p. 94.

13. Michele Cohen, "Rookies in the Cockpit," *News/Sun-Sentinel,* May 22, 1988, pp. 1A+, SIRS, Vol.3, Article No. 69, pp. 7, 8; Collisions and Incursions, op. cit.; "Safety Board Faults Flight Crew in Turboprop Accident at New Orleans," *Air Line Pilot,* August 1988, p. 48.

14. Lori Sharn, "Pilots Blame Errors on Mergers," *USA Today,* November 21, 1989, p. 3A.

15. Anonymous reports from flight crew union officers.

16. Jo Ellen Davis and Pete Engardio, "What It's Like to Work for Frank Lorenzo," *Business Week,* May 18, 1987, pp. 76-78; To Ensure Fair Treatment of Airline Employees in Airline Mergers and Similar Transactions, Hearing Before the Subcommittee on Aviation of the Committee on Public Works and Transportation, House of Representatives, 99th Congress, Second Session on HR 4836 and HR 3838, U.S. Govt. Printing Office, Washington, D.C., 1986.

17. Report from Virginia Technical University, available from the author.

18. Anonymous reports from pilots; Lori Sharn, "Pilots Blame Errors on Mergers," op. cit.; Merger bill HR 4836-3838, op. cit.

19. NOVA television series, "Why Planes Crash," op. cit.

20. Captain W. J. Price and D.C. Holley, Ph.D., "Abnormal Sleep Reduction: A Possible Contributor to the Crash of Pacific Southwest Airlines (PSA) Flight 182," Dept. of Biological Sciences, San Jose State University, San Jose, CA, 1982, pp. 1-10; Holley and Price, "The Probable Contribution of Changing Work/Sleep Schedules in: The Crash of Western Airlines (WAL-Now Delta) Flight 2605 Mexico City, October 31, 1979," Dept. of Biological Sciences, San Jose State University, San Jose, CA, 1982, pp. 4, 5, 9; D.C. Holley, "Circadian Desynchronization and the Sleep-Wake Cycle," pp. 1-10, available from the Dept. of Biological Sciences, San Jose State Univ., San Jose, CA; Conversation between the author and the Los Angeles Disaster Control personnel, 1987; "Pilot Fatigue and Circadian Desynchronosis," report of a workshop held in San Francisco, CA, August 26-28, 1980, NASA Ames Research Center, Moffett Field, CA, 94035, pp. 1-11; Holley and Price, "The Last Minute of Flight 2860: An Analysis of Crew Shift Work Scheduling," Dept. of Biological Sciences, San Jose State University, San Jose, CA, pp. 292-293.

21. Captain W. J. Price and D.C. Holley, Ph.D. "Abnormal Sleep Reduction," op. cit., pp. 1-10; Author's phone conversation with Captain W.J. Price,

1985; Anonymous reports from pilots.

22. "New Approaches to Pilot Training Stress Human Factors, Coordination," *Boston-Aviation Week & Space Technology,* October 16, 1989, pp. 86, 87.

23. "High Accident Rate Continues to Plague Medical Helicopters," *PATA Newsletter,* (Professional Aeromedical Transport Assn.), January 1987, pp. 5, 6.

24. Anthony Broderick letter to Rep. Richardson, op. cit.

25. "In His Own Words," *People Weekly,* op. cit.

26. William Stockton, "Trouble in the Cockpit," *New York Times Magazine,* March 27, 1988, pp. 39, 63; Josef Hebert, "Newest Generation of 'Glass Cockpits' Putting Computers in the Pilot's Seat," *Chicago Tribune,* May 5, 1989, Section 6, pp. 1, 2, SIRS, Vol. 3, Article No. 9.

27. Geraldo Rivera TV special, date and network unknown, 1991.

28. Aviation Safety Research Act of 1988, Federal Register, November 3, 1988.

29. J.C. Paterson, W. Sipes, and D.R. Jones, "Psychiatric Diagnoses and Aeromedical Dispositions of Fliers Referred to the USA School of Aerospace Medicine," USAF School of Aerospace Medicine, Brooks AFB, TX 78235.

30. Jan Steenblik, "Reducing Pilot Error: Who Will Take the Lead?", op. cit., pp. 13-18, 25-30; "FAA Sets Interim Flight/Duty Time Limits for Long-Haul Two-Pilot Flag Operations," *Air Line Pilot,* May 1989, pp. 47-52; NOVA, "Why Planes Crash," op. cit.; Jan Steenblik, "Two Pilots One Team," *Air Line Pilot,* August 1988, p. 10; C.V. Glines, "New Rules for Old Issues," op. cit., p. 29; Hans M. Wegman, Bernard Conrad, and Karl E. Klein, "Flight, Flight Duty, and Rest Times: A Comparison Between the Regulations of Different Countries," *Aviat. Space, & Environ. Medicine,* March 1983, pp. 213-217.

31. "Fight Attendant Duty Time Bill is Introduced in Congress," *Air Line Pilot,* November 1988, p. 12.

32. Author's conversations with flight attendants and Union of Flight Attendants (UFA Local #1) Health and Safety Chairperson, Jana Hakrider, 1987-1990; Teri Agins, "Cabin Fever: Flight Attendants' Lot Loses Allure for Some as Pay and Perks Dive," *Wall Street Journal,* Vol. CXVI, No. 61.

33. Jan. W. Steenblik, op. cit. pp. 12-13.

34. Stoller, Gary; "Is Your Laptop Scaring the Pilot?", *Condé Nast Traveler,* 1993, p. 32; Travel Update column, "Pilots Cite Electronic Gadgets' Effect," *International Herald Tribune,* March 16, 1993, p. 2; CBS Evening News with Dan Rather, June 1993.

35. Jeff Klinkenberg, "The Feathery Bullets: Bird-Plane Collisions A Serious Concern," *St. Petersburg Times,* August 11, 1985, pp. 1F, 3F, reprinted in *Social Issues and Resources Series* (SIRS), Vol. 3, Article #14.

CHAPTER 8 - Jet Lag, Sleep Deprivation, and Circadian Desynchronization ✦

1. Charles F. Ehret and Lynn Waller Scanlon, *Overcoming Jet Lag,* (New York: Berkeley Books, 1983) pp. 16-20; Dr. Gay Luce, *Circadian Rhythms,* 1971, pp. 137-139; Harry Nelson, "Finding Ways to Minimize the Effects of Jet Lag," *The Los Angeles Times,* June 30, 1991, p. L28.

2. *Overcoming Jet Lag,* op. cit.; Arbie Dale, *Biorhythm,* (New York: Pocket Books, 1976), pp. 141-153; Klein Wegmann, et. al., "A Model for Prediction of Resynchronization After Time-Zone Flights," *Aviat. Space Environ. Med.,* June 1983; D.C. Holley, et. al., "Effects of Circadian Rhythm Phase Alteration on Physiological and Psychological Variables: Implications to Pilot Performance," NASA Technical Memorandum 81277, available from Dr. Holley at the Department of Biology, San Jose State University, San Jose, CA, 95192; Nola Lewis, "Scientific Notes: Resetting the Human Clock," from an article in *Noetic Sciences Review, Science,* Vol. 244, 1256, 1328-1333, p. 34.

3. John Travolta interview with Princess Di at White House gala, *People* magazine, April 1985.

4. Jane E. Brody, "Scientists Find Ways to Reset Biological Clocks," *New York Times,* Dec. 29, 1993, p. B7.

5. Stephanie Faul, "How to Beat Jet Lag," *AAA Traveler,* April 1993, p. 13.

6. "Ah, Jet Lag," *Modern Maturity,* January 1992, p. 16.

7. Charles F. Ehret and Lynn Waller Scanlon, *Overcoming Jet Lag,* op. cit., pp. 60-63.

8. Stephen Hall, "Beating Jet Lag With a Diet," *Science 83,* Vol. 4, No. 7, September 1983, p. 88; Harry Nelson, "Finding Ways to Minimize the Effects of Jet Lag," op. cit., p. L18; Ronald E. Kotzsch, "Bringing the Sun Indoors," *East-West,* March 1989, p. 51; also based on co-author Ralph Luciani's NASA research.

9. John A. Amaro, "An Ancient Approach to Beating 20th Century Jet Lag," *MPI's Dynamic Chiropractic,* April 1, 1989. pp. 12-16.

10. CNN Television, "Hour Magazine," January 1984; various TV news reports, 1992.

11. D.C. Holley, "Circadian Desynchronization and the Sleep-Wake Cycle," July 1981, paper available from Dr. Holley at the Department of Biology, San Jose State University, San Jose, CA, 95192; "International Aircrew Sleep/Wakefulness Study," *Aviation Space Environmental Medicine,* December 1986, Vol. 57, No. 12, Section II ASEMOG 57 (12, Suppl: B1-B64).

12. D.C. Holley, "Circadian Desynchronization and the Sleep-Wake Cycle," op. cit.; "Time Changes Also Affect Body Clocks," *Los Angeles Times,* Washington Post-distributed series (no date); W.J. Price and D.C. Holley, "Work, Rest, and Pilot Performance," *Professional Pilot,* May 1981, pp. 74-78.

13. Alice A. Bailey, *Esoteric Psychology,* Vol. II (New York: Lucis Publishing Co.,) pp. 493-512.

14. Richard Rhodes, "You Can Direct Your Dreams," *Parade Magazine,* February 19, 1984, p. 10.

15. D.C. Holley, "Circadian Desynchronization and the Sleep-Wake Cycle," op. cit.

16. NASA Technical Memo 81275, "Pilot Fatigue and Circadian Desynchronosis," 1980, available from Dr. Holley at Dept. of Biology, San Jose State University, San Jose, CA. 95192.

17. NASA Technical Memorandum 81275, "Pilot Fatigue and Circadian Desynchronosis," op. cit.; Charles F. Ehret and Lynn Waller Scanlon,

Overcoming Jet Lag, op. cit.; Dwight Dedmon, "Physiological and Psychological Deficiencies of the Airline Flight Attendant," from Assn. of Flight Attendants (AFA) files.

18. D.C. Holley, "Circadian Desynchronization and the Sleep-Wake Cycle," op. cit.

19. Hubertus Strughold, *Your Body Clock,* (New York: Charles Scribners Sons, 1971), p. 67.

20. D.C. Holley, "Circadian Desynchronization and the Sleep-Wake Cycle," op. cit.

21. D.C. Holley, op. cit.; Arbie Dale, *Biorhythm,* op. cit., pp. 79-80; Charles F. Ehret and Lynn Waller Scanlon, *Overcoming Jet Lag,* op. cit., pp. 74.

CHAPTER 9 - Fleet Fatigue: The Clear and Present Danger of Aging Planes ✈

1. David Tarrant and Ed Timms, "Fatigued Aircraft Unsafe at Any Altitude?", *Dallas Morning News,* December 1, 1985, pp. 1B+, SIRS, Vol. 3, Article No. 20, pp. 1-3; James R. Carroll, "Flying in the Face of Good Sense? Geriatric Jets Draw Heavy Fire," *Wichita Eagle-Beacon,* May 22, 1988, pp. 15A+, SIRS, Vol. 3, Article No. 6, pp. 5-7.

2. James R. Carroll, "Flying in the Face of Good Sense?", op. cit.; Laura Parker, "The Aging of America's Jet Set—Decades of Wear and Tear Raise Growing Safety Concerns," *Washington Post* National Weekly Edition, May 16-22, 1988, pp. 29+, SIRS, Vol. 3, Article No. 69, pp. 3-4; Tom Brokaw, CBS "Nightly News Report," May 23, 1989; "New Products to Solve Old Problems," *National Geographic,* December 1989, p. 749.

3. Anthony Broderick letter to Rep. Bill Richardson, op. cit.

4. James R. Carroll, "Flying in the Face of Good Sense?", op. cit., p. 137; Byron Acohido, Elouise Schumacher, Polly Lane, "Are They Too Old to Fly?", *Seattle Times/Post Intelligencer,* June 19, 1988; David Tarrant and Ed Timms, "Fatigued Aircraft Unsafe at Any Altitude?", op. cit.

5. James R. Carroll, "Flying in the Face of Good Sense?", op. cit., pp. 6-7; David Tarrant and Ed Timms, "Fatigued Aircraft Unsafe at Any Altitude?", op. cit., pp. 1B+, SIRS, pp. 2, 3; *Encyclopedia of Aviation,* (New York: Charles Scribner's Sons, 1977), p. 128.

6. James R. Carroll, "Flying in the Face of Good Sense," op. cit.

7. Tom Webb, "When is a Jet Too Old to Fly? Experts Unsure," *Boca Raton News,* from the KNT newswire, June 5, 1988, p. 2A.

8. Tom Webb, op. cit., p. 2A; James R. Carrol, "Flying in the Face of Good Sense," op. cit., pp. 1B+, SIRS, pp. 1-3; *USA Today,* December 5, 1989; various TV news reports, 1989-92.

9. Brian Ross, *Dateline NBC,* May 5, 1992; *60 Minutes,* CBS, May 19, 1990; Andy Pasztor, "McDonnell Used Substandard Rivets in Air Force Planes, Ex-Employee Says," *The Wall Street Journal* (no date); "Year later, jet crash haunts investigators," *The Washington Post,* (no date).

10. James P. Sterba, "Airborne Acid Proves Costly For Carriers," *The Wall Street Journal,* December 5, 1983, p. 33.

CHAPTER 10 - Healthier Flying: Helpful Hints for Frequent Fliers and Crew Members ✈

1. Joseph D. Alter and Stanley R. Mohler, "Preventative Medicine Aspects and Health Promotion Programs for Flight Attendants," *Aviation, Space and Environmental Medicine,* February 1980, p. 171.

2. Sheldon C. Deal, *New Life through Nutrition,* (Tuscon: New Life Publishing, 1974), pp. 107-116.

3. Lisa Yates' statement, op. cit., Janis S. Bumgarner, Director of Air Safety, AFA, testimony S. 197, November 9, 1983.

4. *Prevention Magazine,* November 1983, Rodale Press, pp. 73-78.

5. Weyling Eng, "Survey on Eye Comfort in Aircraft: 1. Flight Attendants," op. cit., pp. 401-404.

6. UFA Local No. 1. Committee Report, "Health Effects of the Airplane Environment," Vol. IV, No. 4, June 1977.

7. Information on hearing specialists in your area can be obtained by contacting Health Research Group, 2000 P. St. N.W., Suite 708, Washington, D.C. 20036, (202) 842-0320; "Noise: The Universal Menace," *Lifelines: OCAW Health and Safety News,* OCAW Health and Safety Office, Denver, CO, Vol. 1, No. 8, June 1974.

8. Union of Flight Attendants, UFA Local No. 1, Committee Report, "Health Effects of the Airline Environment: Noise. Are You Being Exposed to Too Much?", pp. 1-9; "Noise: the Universal Menace," op. cit.; Aage R. Moller, "Noise As a Health Hazard," *Environmental Health,* pp. 790-791.

9. J. Myers, K. Swenson, L. Kazarian, M. Souder, K. Smith, L. Muhic, R. Cooper, S. Smith, P. Roberts, "Whole-Body Vibration Effects on Calcium Metabolism: A Potential Weightlessness Countermeasure," Wright State University, University of Dayton Research Inst., Dayton, OH 45401-0927; K. Swenson, L. Kazarian, J. Myers, S. Smith, and M. Souder, "The Effects of Low Frequency Vibration on Vertebral Strength," Wright State University, University of Dayton Research Inst., Dayton, OH 45401-0927.

10. Howard D. Kurland, *Back Pains—Quick Relief Without Drugs,* (New York: Simon and Schuster, 1982), pp. 167-168.

11. Toshitada, et. al., "Effects of Relative Metabolic Rate Variation on the Performance of Flight Attendants," *Aviation, Space, and Environmental Medicine,* February 1982, pp. 127-129.

12. "HEAT," OSHA, UFA Committee copy, date unknown; Dr. Richard L. Masters and Dr. William E. Winter, "Flying and Pregnancy," UFA Committee copy; Statements made by Dr. Kenneth Lyon Jones at the ASMA meeting, May 1987.

13. For further information contact: "Nutra Sweet," CBS News, Virginia Beach, VA 23463, or contact Dr. John Olne at Washington University in St. Louis.

14. "Continuum," *OMNI,* February 1988, p. 37.

15. Don and Julia Downie, "Oxygen Breathes New Life into Performance," *Private Pilot,* October 1984, p. 16.

16. Author's conversations with Captain Andy Yates and other crew members.

17. Jane Briggs-Bunting, et. al., "Here I was Sitting at the Edge of Eternity," *Life,* March 1989, pp. 29+; Laurie McGinley, "Fear of Landing—A Flight Attendant, DC-10 Crash Survivor Struggles to Come Back," *Wall Street Journal,* Vol. CCXV, No. 13.

18. Former EAL chairman, anonymous.

CHAPTER 11 - Stress in the Skies and How to Cope With It ✈

1. Stewart Powell with Marilyn A. Moore and Sharon F. Golden, "A Sick and Tired Pilot Who Had Enough," *U.S. News and World Report,* December 22, 1986, pp. 14+, SIRS, Vol. 3, Article No. 40, pp. 2-3.

2. "The FAA's Sweat Shops," *Washington Post,* op. cit., pp. 1-3.

3. For detailed information about stress and its effects, I suggest reading: *Stress Without Distress,* Hans Selye, (New York: Signet, 1974); *The Stress of Life,* Hans Selye, (New York: McGraw Hill, 1956); *Stress Management for Chronic Disease,* Michael Russel, (Pergamon, 1988); Alan S. Dietz, "Biochemical Events During Stress," *Anabolism, Journal of Preventative Medicine,* Vol. 1, No. 1, August 1982, pp. 9-10; *Recovering from the War,* Patience Mason.

4. Hans Selye, *Stress Without Distress,* op. cit.; Hans Selye, *The Stress of Life,* op. cit.; Alan S. Dietz, "Biochemical Events During Stress," op. cit., pp. 9, 10; Stephen A. Levine and Parris M. Kidd, "Antioxidant Adaptation: A Unified Disease Theory," *J. Orthomolecular Psychiatry,* Vol. 14, No. 1, First Quarter, 1985; pp. 19-24, Larry Slonaker, "Airplane 1988—A Disaster Story," *East-West,* April 24, 1988.

5. James E. Crane, B.S., M.D., D.A.S. (HON), FAA Sr. Flight Surgeon, "Light and Stress," *Healthline—Aviation Medicine and Physical Fitness,* Vol. 1, No. 1, July 1984, p. 6; *East-West,* op. cit., p. 51.

6. "Meditate Your Way to Staying Younger," *Prevention,* p. 116, (date unknown), source, *Int. Neuroscience,* Vol. 16, No. 1, pp. 53-57; "Laughing Toward Longevity," *University of California-Berkeley Wellness Letter,* June 1985, published in association with the School of Public Health.

CHAPTER 12 - Inflight Emergencies and Passenger Survival ✈

1. S. 197, September 19, 1986, op. cit.

2. "Special Report: U.S. Airlines in Crisis," Travel & Leisure, December 1993, p. 180.

3. For more information about emergency survival see Daniel A. Johnson, *Just in Case,* purchase c/o President, Interactions Research Corp., Olympia, WA; Videos and training courses are provided by Stark Survival Co. in Panama City, FL.

4. Dr. H. Beau Altman and Dr. Daniel A. Johnson, The Interaction Research Corp., "Aircraft Passenger Safety: Passenger Education and Survival,"

UFA Committee Copy, p. 14.

5. "Safety First," *Parade Magazine,* August 25, 1985, p. 21.

6. "Some Examples of Just What the Passenger is Agreeing to," *New York Times,* January 28, 1990; Bob Maynard, Universal Press, "Air Travel: Rules for Flying While Waiting for Disaster," *The (Santa Fe) New Mexican,* October 10, 1987.

7. Joseph D. Younger, *AAA World,* November/December 1990, pp. 10-12.

8. Mary Johnson, Editor of the Disability Rag, "Enabling Act," *The Nation,* October 23, 1989, p. 446.

9. Carole Jacobs, "Knowing Where It's Safe to Travel Overseas," *Vacation,* Winter 1991, p. 51-53.

CHAPTER 13 - How to Be Fit For Flying Through Proper Nutrition →

1. Rudolph Ballentine, Diet and Nutrition, (Homesdale, PA: The Himalayan International Institute, 1978), pp. 7-10; various news media reports 1980-92.

2. Henry G. Bieler, *Food is Your Best Medicine,* (New York: Vintage, 1973), pp. 208-213; Abram Hoffer, "Nutrition and Behavior," *Medical Application of Clinical Nutrition,* Jeffrey Bland, ed., (New Canaan, CT: Keats Publishing, 1983), pp. 238-241.

3. Robert C. Atkins, *Dr. Atkins' Diet Revolution,* (New York: Bantam Books, 1972); Jeffrey Bland, *Your Health Under Siege: Using Nutrition to Fight Back,* (Battleboro, VT: Stephen Greene Press, 1981); Colin H. Dong and Jane Banks, *New Hope for the Arthritic,* (New York: Thomas Y. Crowell, 1975); Henry G. Bieler, *Food is Your Best Medicine,* op. cit.; Max Gerson, *A Cancer Therapy,* (Del Mar, CA: Totality Books, Third Ed., 1977).

4. For further information, contact Dr. William Donald Kelley, International Health Institute, P.O. Box 402607, Dallas, Texas, 75240; Roger J. Williams, *Biochemical Individuality,* (Austin: University of Texas Press, 1975); George Watson, *Personality Strength and Psycho-Chemical Energy,* (New York: Harper & Row, 1979); Sheldon C. Deal, *New Life Through Nutrition,* op. cit., pp. 128-139; Jeffrey Bland, "Blood Sugar Problems and Late 20th Century Living," *Your Health Under Siege,* op. cit., pp. 168-174.

5. Frances Moore Lappe, *Diet for a Small Planet,* (New York: Friends of the Earth, 1971); Ellen Buchman Ewald, *Recipes for a Small Planet,* (New York: Ballantine Books, 1973).

6. Nathan Pritikin and Patrick M. McGrady, Jr., *The Pritikin Program for Diet and Exercise,* (New York: Grosset and Dunlap, 1979), p. 5.

7. John D. Kirschmann, *Nutrition Almanac,* Revised Ed., (New York: McGraw-Hill Book Company, 1979), revised each year; Rudolph Ballentine, *Diet and Nutrition,* op. cit., p. 141; Frances Moore Lappe, *Diet for a Small Planet,* op. cit., p. 42.

8. James F. Balch, & Phyllis A. Balch, *Prescription for Nutritional Healing,* (New York: Avery Publishing Group Inc., 1990).

9. Jeffrey Bland, *Your Health Under Siege,* op. cit., p. 243; Ross Hume Hall, *Food For Nought,* (New York: Vintage, 1976).

10. David Stipp,"Studies Showing Benefits of Antioxidants," *Wall Street Journal,* April 13, 1993, p. B1.

11. William H. Philpott and Dwight K. Kalita, *Brain Allergies,* (New Canaan, CT: Keats Publishing, 1980), p. 60.

12. Supplemental suggestions are mostly summarized from Carl C. Pfeiffer's *Mental and Elemental Nutrients,* New Canaan, CT: Keats Publishing, 1980, pp. 95, 115-125.

13. Richard A. Passwater, "L-Glutamine, The Surprising Brain Fuel," *Health Express,* Vol. 2, No. 6, August 1981, pp. 8-11.

14. Dirk Pearson and Sandy Shaw, *Life Extension,* New York: Warner Books, 1980, p. 131.

15. Marcia Holly, "Body Timing: Clock Your Real, Not Phony, Rhythms," Health Watch 2, *Self,* July 1982, p. 22.

16. Eugene C. Olinete, M.D., "The Royal Jelly Story," 7171 Mercy Rd., Suite 135, Omaha, NB 68106.

17. Dr. Schulesoler, "Cell Salts," Standard Homeopathic Co., PO Box 61067, Los Angeles, CA, 90061.

18. Rudolph Ballentine, *Diet and Nutrition,* op. cit., pp. 7-10; Jeffrey Bland, *Your Health Under Siege:,* op. cit., p. 243.

19. Beers, Kenneth N. and Mohler, Stanely R., "Food Poisoning as an In-Flight Safety Hazard," *Aviation, Space and Environmental Medicine,* June 1985.

20. Kathleen Doheney, "Cholera Represents a Distant but Real Danger," *Los Angeles Times,* March 22, 1992.

CHAPTER 14 - What Is (and Isn't) Being Done to Make Flying Safer and Healthier ✈

1. Smoking Ban, HR 2040, op. cit.; statement by Senator Inouye, S. 2746, "The Aviation Safety Research Act of 1988," Senate Commerce Committee, September 20, 1988, Executive Session.

2. Lori Sharn, "FAA Not Flying by its Own Rules," *USA Today,* Nov. 26, 1993.p. 2.

3. *USA Today* (international edition), April 28, 1993; p. 8A.

4. "Deregulation a Mistake, Former Congressional Supporter Says," *Air Line Pilot,* January 1988, p. 38; Tom Eblen, "Airline Deregulation: Bane to Some, Boon to Many," *Atlanta Journal & Constitution,* October 9, 1988; Paul Stephen Dempsey, *Flying Blind: The Failure of Airline Deregulation,* Economic Policy Institute, 1730 Rhode Island Ave. N.W., Suite 812, Washington D.C. 20036, ISBN 0-944826-23-7, 1990, p. 2-3, 23, 60.

5. Julie Schmit, "Holiday Fliers Take Off," *USA Today,* November 23, 1993, pp. 1-2.

6. David Tarrant and Ed Timms, "Fatigued Aircraft Unsafe at any Altitude?", *Dallas Morning News,* op. cit., p. 1; James Carrol, "Flying in the Face of Good Sense: Geriatric Jets Draw Heavy Fire," *Wichita Eagle-Beacon,* op. cit.

7. "The Federal Aviation Administration's Airline Safety Inspection Program," Hearings Before the Subcommittee on Aviation of the Committee on Public Works and Transportation, House of Representatives, 99th Congress, 2nd

Session, May 14, 15, and 22, 1986, U.S. Govt. Printing Office, Washington D.C., 1986, pp. 1, 3, 5-12; *NBC Morning News*, 3/22/90, 3/28/90.

8. Anthony Broderick letter to Rep. Bill Richardson, op. cit., 1993.

9. "The Effects of the President's Budget and Gramm-Rudman-Hollings on Aviation Programs," Hearing Before the Subcomm. on Aviation of the Comm. on Public Works and Transportation, House of Representatives, 99th Congress, 2nd Session, Mar. 12, 1986, opening statement by Rep. Norman Mineta, pp. 1-7; "Aviation Safety" (Status of the U.S. Air Traffic Control System), Hearing Before the Subcomm. on Investigations and Oversight, Committee on Public Works and Transportation, 101st Congress, 1st Session, May 25, 1989, U.S. Government Printing Office, Washington D.C., 1989, pp. 1-3, 7, 56; "Near Midair Collisions and Runway Incursions," Hearing Before the Subcomm. on Investigation and Oversight, Aviation Safety, Comm. on Public Works and Transportation, House of Representatives, 100th Congress, 1st Session, April 9, 1987, Testimony in entirety, U.S. Government Printing Office, Washington D.C., 1988.

10. "Near Midair Collisions and Runway Incursions," op. cit., pp. 30-32; Broderick letter to Rep. Richardson, op. cit.

11. Smoking Ban, HR 2040 op. cit.; Statement by Sen. Inouye, S. 2746, "The Aviation Safety Research Act of 1988," op. cit.

12. Federal Aviation Administration (FAA) Advisory Committee for Radiation Biology Aspects for the Super Sonic Transport (SST), 1975, "Final Report, Cosmic Radiation Exposure in Supersonic and Subsonic Flight," *Aviation Space Environmental Medicine,* p. 46, 117.

13. Broderick letter to Rep. Richardson, op. cit.

14. ibid.

15. ibid.

16. "Schedule for Installation of the TCAS-II Collision Avoidance System," Report (to accompany HR 2151) by Rep. Glenn M. Anderson, from the Committee on Public Works and Transportation, 101st Congress, 1st Session, House of Representatives, Report 101-174, July 26, 1989, pp. 1-3; *NBC News,* 3/28/90, op. cit. Broderick letter to Rep. Richardson, op. cit.

17. Broderick letter to Rep. Richardson, op. cit.

18. "Impact of International Terrorism on Travel," Joint Hearings Before the Subcommittee on Arms Control, International Operations of the Committee on Foreign Affairs and the Subcommittee on Aviation of the Committee on Public Works and Transportation, 99th Congress, 2nd Session, February 19, April 17, 22, and May 15, 1986, U.S. Government Printing Office, Washington D.C., 1986, p. 290; "Aviation Security," Hearings Before the Subcommittee on Aviation of the Committee on Public Works and Transportation, House of Representatives, 101st Congress, 1st Session, March 21, 1989 and April 25, 1989, pp. 53-55, 147, 149, 151, 152, 225, 226.

19. Broderick letter to Rep. Richardson, op. cit.; Federal Register, "Explosive Detection Systems: Notice of Proposed Criteria for Certification," November 4, 1992.